# EDUCATION
# 4KNEES©

EVERYTHING
YOU NEED TO KNOW
FOR HAPPY, HEALTHY AND
PAIN-FREE KNEES

GREGORY M. MARTIN, M.D.

WITH A

10 MINUTE-A-DAY KNEE FITNESS PROGRAM
BY BOB HABIB, RPT

# DEDICATION

To my patients: they have educated me more
than I have educated them. This book is my way
of giving back.
To my wife Patty, my children Madison & Max, and my
entire extended family: knowing the love and support a
family can provide has enabled me to be compassionate
and recognize the importance of decision making when
it comes to our health. As a knee surgeon, I often get
asked "what would you recommend if I was a member of
your family?"........This book answers that question.

StarGroup International, Inc. West Palm Beach, Florida

Supervision: Brenda Star

Book design: Mel Abfier

Cover design: Sandor Valdes

Senior Editor: Gwen Carden

Proofreaders: Edie Tall, Linda Haase

Designed and produced by StarGroup International, Inc.
(561) 547-0667
www.stargroupinternational.com

Printed in the United States of America

Library of Congress Control Number: 2013955980

EDUCATION 4KNEES
ISBN 978-1-884886-65-2

The information contained within EDUCATION4KNEES is not intended or implied to be a substitute for professional medical advice, diagnosis or treatment. All content, including text, graphics, images and, information contained within this book are for general information purposes only. EDUCATION4KNEES does not recommend, endorse or make any representation about the efficacy, appropriateness or suitability of any specific tests, products, procedures, treatments, services, opinions, health care providers or other information that may be contained within this book. The author and publisher are not responsible or liable for any advice, course of treatment, diagnosis or any other treatment, services or products you obtain as a result of reading this book. You are encouraged to confirm any information obtained from or through this book with other sources, and review all information regarding any medical condition or treatment with your physician.

Never disregard professional medical advice or delay seeking medical treatment because of something you read in this book. The reader should regularly consult a physician in all matters relating to his or her health, particularly in respect to any symptoms that may require diagnosis or medical attention.

# TABLE OF CONTENTS

# INTRODUCTION

Do your knees crack when you walk? Has it become excrutiating to make it through all nine holes of your usual golf game? Do you wonder when or if that pain is really going to go away?

Whether I'm at a party with friends or attending an outing at my children's school, someone always wants to talk to me about their aching knees. There's the retiree who has stopped going out to dinner with friends because it's too painful to walk from the parking lot to the restaurant. There are parents who can't take their kids to Disney World — all that standing and waiting in line is too much to even think about! There's the tennis fanatic who hasn't been on the court in ages. And then there are unfortunate ones who can't even work or go up and down stairs without discomfort. The stories are varied, but all reflect people's frustrations at not being able to do what they want to do. It isn't just grandparents approaching me with knee ailments. Many are in fact young adults. One of these stories might even sound like yours.

Whether you're suffering from occasional aches, arthritis or any other type of knee pain, or you're just trying to avoid future knee problems, this book is for you. The treatments you'll read about can help anyone from an 18-year-old ballet dancer to a weekend warrior to a 90-year-old with arthritis, and everyone in between.

I'm drawing from my experience dealing with thousands of patients with every degree of pain and discomfort, so I know what works. And more importantly, what doesn't. After reading this book, you will know what's causing those creaky knees, that twinge when you turn suddenly, the shooting pain when you simply try to climb the stairs.

I share this information to cut through the confusion, and because it's so important—almost everyone's knees will give them trouble eventually. Sure, there are other resources available, but they're usually filled with medical jargon and extraneous information that bores even me, an orthopedic surgeon. While this is not intended to be a comprehensive resource for knee pain, it will provide an overview of what you need to know about knee pain and how to avoid it. I've eliminated the clutter and boiled the information down to what will make you feel better, improve your life and minimize or eliminate your discomfort. If something isn't mentioned, it's because I don't believe it is helpful or there is not enough evidence to support its use.

The result: an easy-to-understand road map that will tell you how to keep your knees healthy – and what to do if they start to ache. The treatments and options included are designed to avoid or postpone surgery while eliminating or reducing pain. If surgery is required, the information provided will help you achieve the best possible outcome. My suggestions are designed to fit into your busy and active life.

Keep in mind that there is no magic solution, but there is a simple solution. It involves creating a lifestyle to make your knees feel as good as possible.

Each chapter offers easy-to-use tips and detailed illustrations, along with highlighted summaries, to guide you through what you need to know.  Chapters 1 through 3 will teach you about the anatomy of the knee, what can go wrong, and why modern medicine and surgery don't solve many people's knee problems. Chapters 4 through 8 will introduce a 4-part lifestyle solution that anyone can follow and get their knees feeling great.  Chapter 9 discusses what you can do when, despite doing the things in Chapters 4 through 8, the knee still has a problem.  Chapter 10 will then bring it all together.

So, sit back, put your feet up and let's get started. No co-pay required.

P.S.  A personal note: My father and grandfather were auto repairmen, and growing up, I spent a lot of time working or hanging around in their shop. You may notice several times in the book that I compare what is going on with the knee to a similar situation in a car. It just comes naturally to me and, besides, I think those sorts of analogies can help someone without a medical background more easily understand difficult concepts. The knee doesn't have to be so complicated, and that's why I'm excited to bring you this book.

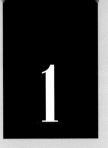

# OVERVIEW OF KNEE ANATOMY

What you will learn in this chapter:

• The knee is one of the largest and most complex joints in your body

• The knee is made up of three bones

• The knee joint is made up of three parts

• Cartilage is the lining of the knee joint and is crucial because it allows pain-free motion

• Joint fluid, the lubricant of the knee, helps prevent friction

• The main muscles around the knee are the quadriceps and hamstrings, which coordinate to enable you to walk, run and jump

• Other important components of the knee are tendons and ligaments, as well as nerves and blood vessels

When I was in my first year of college, I was unsure of exactly what I wanted to do with my life. I had no background in science and there were no doctors in my family. I never thought about my knee or any of my joints. I was young and nothing hurt me. That all changed one day after an unfortunate accident where I fell through a window and a giant piece of glass lacerated my right leg just above my kneecap. I learned two important things that day; first, what my knee looks like on the inside and second, that I wanted to be a surgeon to help as many people as I could (just like the doctor who helped sew my leg back together). I changed my major to pre-med and the rest is history.

This book is part of my quest to help as many people as possible. The first task at hand, learning some of the basic anatomy, is perhaps the least interesting for some people. It is, however, important for understanding what is normal and what can go wrong. I will try and simplify it as much as possible so you don't have to get an "inside view" as I did in college.

We all know what a knee looks like on the outside, but when it comes to using it, it's what you don't see that's important.

Your knee may look small, but it's one of the largest and most complex joints in your body.

The knee is what is known as a "hinge joint." Think of it like a car door – opening and closing dozens of times a week (only the knee moves thousands of times a week). Like the door, it can start to creak after years of use, and there's no WD-40 to get it back into good working order. Also, like a car door hinge, it's connected by an intricate system that's easy to take for granted until it breaks.

# HERE IS WHAT YOU NEED TO KNOW
## ABOUT THE STRUCTURES
## THAT MAKE UP THE KNEE

## KNEE BONES

The knee is composed of three bones:
Femur (thigh bone)
Tibia (shin bone)
Patella (kneecap)

The bottom of the femur, the top of the tibia, and the backside of the patella make up the knee joint.

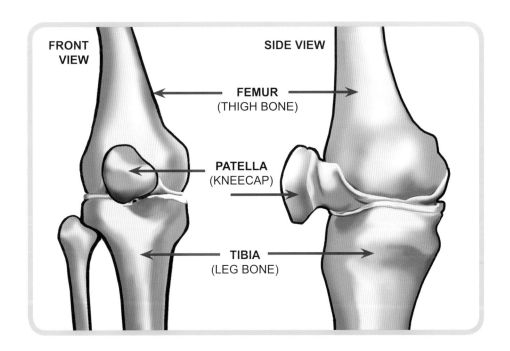

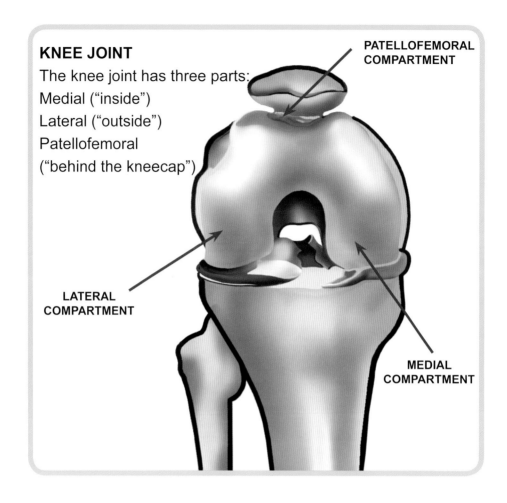

**KNEE JOINT**

The knee joint has three parts:

Medial ("inside")

Lateral ("outside")

Patellofemoral

("behind the kneecap")

PATELLOFEMORAL
COMPARTMENT

LATERAL
COMPARTMENT

MEDIAL
COMPARTMENT

## CARTILAGE

All knees contain cartilage, which acts as lining for the ends of all of our joints. Cartilage is a soft, spongy, tissue found in many parts of the body including the nose, ear, rib cage, the air tubes to the lungs and spine. It's harder than muscle but softer than bone.

Cartilage is a crucial structure in the knee because it enables pain-free motion as you walk, run and bend. It's unlike most other tissues of the body in three important ways:

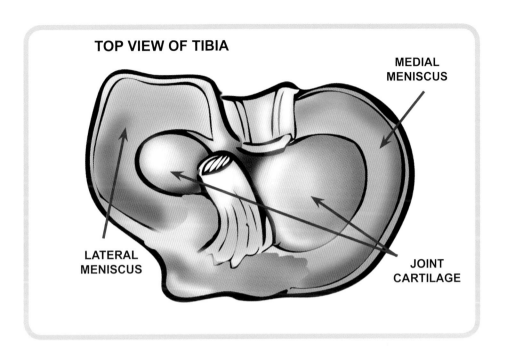

**TOP VIEW OF TIBIA**

MEDIAL MENISCUS

LATERAL MENISCUS

JOINT CARTILAGE

It is comprised mostly of water, it has no nerve supply, and it has a poor blood supply.

What does this mean for the knee?

When hydrated properly, cartilage is composed of up to 80 percent water, which is typical in younger people. As a person ages, the water content can drop to as low as 70 percent. Drinking lots of water is one key to good knee health and will be covered later.

Cartilage has no nerve endings. Nerves are what lead to the sensation of pain. In a healthy knee, cartilage rubs against cartilage and no pain is felt. If cartilage breaks down, nerve endings in the bone become exposed and sensitive, leading to pain.

Because cartilage has a very poor blood supply – reaching only to its edges - there are no blood vessels to carry nutrients into it.

Only movement helps achieve this function. Therefore, maintaining movement in your knees is crucial to keeping cartilage alive and healthy.

Poor blood supply subjects the knee cartilage to limited ability to heal – thus making preservation of the cartilage a major goal.

There are two types of cartilage found in the knee joint.

## MENISCUS CARTILAGE

The knee has two C-shaped disks called the lateral meniscus (on the outside of the knee) and the medial meniscus (on the inside of the knee) Located between the femur and tibia, they cushion and reduce friction between the two sides of the knee joint and work like shock absorbers when walking or running.   The main role of the meniscal cartilage is to protect the joint cartilage.

## JOINT CARTILAGE

Joint cartilage, called articular cartilage, is a slick, white substance that covers the ends of the bones of the knee. It permits smooth movement of the bones with minimal friction. Joint cartilage is more durable than meniscus cartilage and thus more difficult to injure. However, whenever two surfaces rub against each other, it leads to friction and wear (just like the tires of your car wear from touching the road).  So over time this cartilage can wear away.

## LUBRICATION AND CAPSULE

Although you can't see or feel it, your knees are filled with fluid which acts as a lubricant and contributes to less friction on (and damage to) the cartilage. If there's too little of it, the joint moves painfully or not at all.  If there is too much, it also creates pain by stretching the joint.

The knee is surrounded by a bag like structure called the capsule. The capsule contains the fluid and bathes the joint in the fluid.

## LIGAMENTS

Ligaments are tough bands of tissue that support or strengthen joints by connecting bone to bone. Their main use is to keep the bones in alignment and provide for a stable joint.

There are 4 major ligaments inside the knee.
Medial collateral ligament (MCL) on the inside.
Lateral collateral ligament (LCL) on the outside.
Anterior cruciate ligament (ACL), which crosses in the middle of the joint in the front.
Posterior cruciate ligament (PCL), which crosses in the middle of the joint in the back.

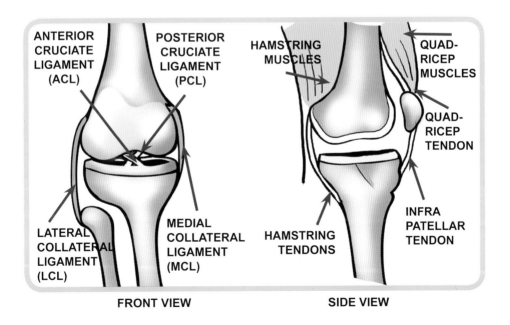

FRONT VIEW          SIDE VIEW

# MUSCLES

The most important muscles surrounding the knee are called the quadriceps (in the front of the thigh) and the hamstrings (in the back of the thigh). When these two major muscle groups are coordinating, you're able to walk, run, and jump.

The quadriceps connects through the quadriceps tendon to the patella. The patella then connects to the tibia via the infrapatellar tendon. This is called the extensor mechanism, which is responsible for straightening the leg.

The hamstrings are a group of muscles and tendons that cross the back of the knee and are responsible for flexing the knee.

# TENDONS

Tendons are elastic tissues that are technically part of the muscle. They connect muscles to bones and help stabilize the knee. The two major tendon structures in the knee are the extensor mechanism (quadriceps tendon and the patellar tendon) in the front of the knee and the hamstring tendons in the back of the knee.

## Other Important Parts

There are numerous other parts that are critical. These include healthy nerves which travel all the way down from the brain through the back (in the spinal cord) and healthy blood vessels which carry oxygen and nutrients to and away from the knee.

When all these parts are functioning properly, we don't even think about our knees, but when they aren't we get reminders all day long.

Next, we'll talk about what can go wrong in the knee.

# 2

# WHY (MOST) KNEES GO BAD

What you will learn in this chapter:

• The knee is a complex joint, and there are a lot of things that can go wrong

• For most adults, it usually doesn't matter why knees go bad – many of the best treatments will often be the same

• Problems that can occur include various forms of arthritis, meniscal tears, cysts in the back of the knee, pain behind the kneecap, and trauma to the knee bones, ligaments, and tendons. Other problems can be caused by a Baker's cyst (a.k.a popliteal cyst), effusions or patellofemoral pain syndrome/chondromalacia

• There can be some very serious causes of knee pain like infections and tumors, but these are rare

• Knee pain can also arise from areas of the body outside of the knee

As you just learned in Chapter 1, the knee has a lot of important structures, so you can imagine there is a lot that can go wrong. Before I talk to you about the most common reasons that knees go bad, however, I want to tell you something that may surprise you: **"In most cases for adults, despite what is going on inside the knee, the best initial treatments are going to be the same."** These treatments, if implemented, can help postpone or possibly even avoid the need for surgery. If surgery is required these same treatments, if continued, will help ensure the best possible outcome.

> *"If surgery is required, the same treatments will ensure the best possible outcome."*

You're probably wondering how can that be possible? How is it that your neighbor's treatment for his meniscus tear could by any stretch of the imagination be the same as the treatment for your arthritic knee?

Glad you asked. The short answer is that there is a "final common pathway" for most knee problems in adults. We will get to that in Chapter 3, but first let's define the most common issues and problems we encounter in the knee. These include:

1. Types of arthritis
2. Meniscal tears
3. Baker's cyst (popliteal cyst)
4. Patellofemoral pain syndrome/chondromalacia ("runner's knee")
5. Trauma to the knee leading to fractures, inflammation or ligament or tendon ruptures
6. Other issues

# TYPES OF ARTHRITIS

After diagnosing patients with arthritis in their knee, many will often exclaim in disbelief, "It's just arthritis?" It seems like they are almost disappointed that it wasn't something more serious, or they don't believe that arthritis is capable of causing such a problem.

Well, the complete opposite is true. Arthritis is one of the leading causes of disability in the United States, and there are several forms of it that most commonly impact knee health.

# OSTEOARTHRITIS

The vast majority of people who come to see me have pain because of osteoarthritis (OA), also called degenerative joint disease. OA, the form of arthritis most commonly associated with aging, is caused by the wearing away of the cartilage that covers the knee joint, resulting in the bones being exposed and rubbing together. No one knows for sure why this happens. It appears to be a combination of wear and tear, genetics, aging, and other factors such as weight, prior injury to the knee and limb alignment. Osteoarthritis can be primary, meaning we are not sure why the knee wore out, or secondary to (meaning caused by) another condition such as obesity, prior meniscus injury or surgery or previous fracture. This is an important point to understand as we talk about the final common pathway for our knees.

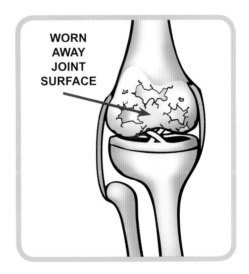

*A knee joint with osteoarthritis.*

*Xray of a normal knee joint and one with osteoarthritis.*

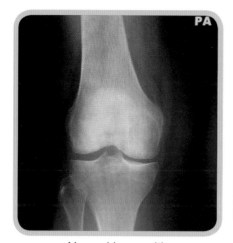 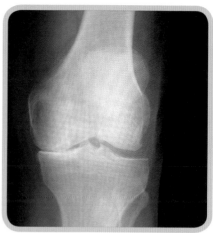

*Normal knee with healthy joint space*

*Arthritic knee with loss of joint space, "Bone on Bone"*

## RHEUMATOID AND OTHER FORMS OF INFLAMMATORY ARTHRITIS

Another type of arthritis that can affect the knees is inflammatory arthritis. Although the symptoms in the knee can appear similar to those caused by OA, the cause of knee pain with inflammatory arthritis such as rheumatoid arthritis (RA) is radically different. RA is a disease that activates the body's immune system to attack itself, mistaking healthy cells, including those that line the joints, for invaders. This attack results in inflammation which eventually wears down the cartilage, causing pain and decreased functioning. Inflammatory arthritis is significantly less common than OA. Other causes of inflammatory arthritis include psoriatic arthritis, lupus and gout.

The common aspect of these inflammatory conditions is that there is something systemic that needs to be treated first in order for your knees to have any hope of feeling better. Inflammatory arthritis can lead to secondary degeneration of the joint, especially if not treated.  (In fact, joint replacement surgery used to be much more common in people with rheumatoid arthritis until newer drugs and treatments were able to alter the course of the disease.)

## MENISICAL TEARS

As we learned in Chapter 1, there are two C-shaped, rubbery discs inside the knee called the lateral and medial meniscus.  These can commonly tear.  In a 15-year-old, it will often take a serious injury or trauma to tear a meniscus.  As we age, the meniscus becomes more brittle and can tear from twisting the wrong way or even squatting down to pick up the newspaper.  A torn meniscus can cause pain as well as mechanical symptoms such as locking, catching and buckling.  However,

*"meniscal tears do not always cause pain. In fact, meniscal tears are extremely common in asymptomatic knees (knees that don't have any pain)."*

Because of a lack of blood supply to the meniscal cartilage, these rarely heal.

*Illustration shows a meniscal tear.*

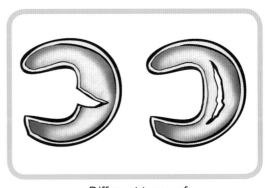

*Different types of Meniscal tears*

# BAKER'S CYST (POPLITEAL CYST) AND EFFUSIONS

A normal amount of joint fluid is healthy and necessary, but if the knee becomes inflamed it can create extra fluid causing what is referred to as an effusion. The extra fluid can stretch the capsule, leading to the sensation of pressure. Sometimes, some of this fluid pushes out the capsule in the back of the knee, leading to a cyst adjacent to the muscle. This is commonly called a Baker's cyst. The cyst itself is not usually the problem. The cyst is typically the result of whatever happened inside the knee to cause the extra fluid.

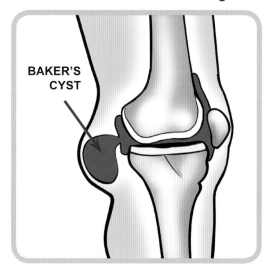

*Illustration shows a Baker's cyst.*

# PATELLOFEMORAL PAIN SYNDROME/ CHONDROMALACIA

Commonly called "runner's knee," this condition can occur in people who put a lot of demands on their knee from excessive running, jumping, bending, squatting or stair climbing. They usually experience pain or aching in the front of the knee. It can be caused by several different factors, but the common aspect is abnormal force on the joint cartilage resulting in discomfort. This leads to thinning or damage to the cartilage called chondromalacia.

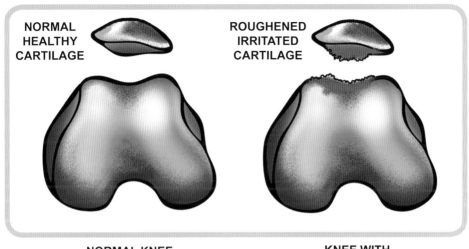

NORMAL KNEE

KNEE WITH
PATELLOFEMORAL
PAIN

## TRAUMA

Injury to the knee can occur as a result of serious trauma such as a fall, car accident or sports injury, or can occur as a result of repetitive small injuries which you may not even be aware of (this is called "microtrauma"). Either way, there are many things that can go wrong and sudden injuries that are severe should always be assessed by an appropriate physician. Fractures can occur which damage the joint surface of the bones around the knee. Ligaments, muscles and tendons can get sprained, strained or torn, partially or completely. Bursitis, tendonitis and other forms of inflammation around the joint can also occur from repetitive irritation or trauma. Combinations of many of the above are also possible.

## OTHER ISSUES

Of course, there are some serious, though rare, causes of knee pain, including infections and tumors that need urgent care, so I always advise patients to never neglect knee pain. If it is severe, persistent or associated with other symptoms, get it checked out.

Also,

*"sometimes the pain being felt in the knee can actually be coming from outside of the knee."*

Problems with the nerves or blood vessels, the lumbar spine, or the hip joint can all lead to pain felt in the knee.......and there may be nothing wrong with the knee itself. This is hard for people to understand, but true in some cases. Mental states, such as anxiety and depression, also play a tremendous role. Although not the direct cause of pain, these conditions impact how pain is perceived and can amplify symptoms (as evidence, the FDA has recently approved an antidepressant for treating arthritis).

Next, let's take a look at what modern medicine can – and cannot – do for your knee pain and learn about the "final common pathway."

# 3

# THE LIMITATIONS OF MODERN MEDICINE
# AND THE FINAL COMMON PATHWAY

What you will learn in this chapter:

- The Final Common Pathway for most knees is degeneration of the joint over time
- Most of the things that can go wrong in the knee can be linked to degenerative joint disease
- The main limitation of modern medicine is that it only looks at the anatomical problems and not the overall picture
- How we treat our knees influences, to some degree, how they wear and how they feel
- Why the knee hurts doesn't really matter most of the time, the initial things that can make it feel better are the same

Now that we understand the common things that can go wrong in the knee, it's time to get back to understanding why for treatment, it doesn't really matter too much in most cases. Let's start with a case example.

Fred, 65, is a recreational tennis player. His knees have been bothering him off and on, but he's ignored the pain. One day he jumps to return a volley, and boom! "Something" pops in his knee, and he's in excruciating pain. The first call is to his wife to come get him. The next is to his doctor.

The doctor takes a "history" (asks Fred a few questions about his health and specific questions about his knee). He conducts an examination, looking for tenderness, swelling, deformity and instability in the knee, then orders an x-ray which shows some early signs of osteoarthritis and then orders an MRI.

Yup. No surprise here. Fred has a tear in his meniscus cartilage and a Baker's cyst visible on MRI. (The reason there is no surprise is because the majority of knees that have an MRI performed in someone like Fred will have some damage to the meniscus and perhaps a Baker's cyst.......even if the person has no pain or symptoms!)

Most likely the doctor is going to order pain medication or an anti-inflammatory, give a cortisone injection and possibly prescribe a short course of physical therapy. When these interventions don't provide Fred permanent relief that enables him to resume his active lifestyle, the doctor will often recommend arthroscopic surgery. Some doctors may even offer arthroscopic surgery right away. Arthroscopic surgery is a technique utilizing a small camera instrument inserted into the knee joint that allows the surgeon to see the joint in great detail on a television monitor.

One problem with rushing to arthroscopic surgery for Fred and for thousands of other people with a similar situation is that in many cases – according to study after study – people are often unhappy with the results.

Another problem is that surgery has risk, and in most cases, should be used after non-operative options fail.

The biggest problem though, and the reason why many patients are not happy after surgery, is that the surgery doesn't address the real cause of the pain in the knee. The meniscus tear and the Baker's cyst are not the cause of Fred's knee pain, they are the result of the knee wearing out.

### THIS IS THE FINAL COMMON PATHWAY.

What I am going to tell you may be a bit controversial, and you may not be happy to hear it.

*"There is a final common pathway for our knees. If we live long enough almost all of our knees will wear out."*

This is called degenerative joint disease. Nearly all of the causes of knee pain that we reviewed in Chapter 2 can be linked to degenerative joint disease. Whenever two surfaces rub together there is friction and wear. If we drive our car, we can't expect there to be no wear on the tires. How long the tires last depends a lot on how they are treated. If an 85-year-old cautious grandma is driving the car, the tires will likely last a lot longer than if an 18-year-old boy is driving. Cars on a racetrack under extreme conditions will wear out their tires quickly. Our knees are no different. How we treat them determines how long they will last, but we can't change the fact that they are wearing. The tires can also wear out quicker if they are made of softer rubber, if there is not enough air in them, if the wheels are out of alignment, if the car is too heavy, if there is previous damage to the treads, etc, etc, etc. What I am getting at is there are a lot of factors that determine the ultimate fate of the tires on our car, but eventually they will all wear out. Our knees are no different!

*Chart below explains different things that can commonly cause knee pain and their link to degenerative joint disease (DJD).*

| | |
|---|---|
| Cartilage Loss/Wear & Tear/Genetics | Leads to DJD which in end stage is "bone on bone" arthritis |
| Meniscal Tears | Almost all knees with DJD have meniscal degeneration and/or tears. Healthy knees with meniscal tears develop DJD at an accelerated rate. |
| Baker's Cyst (Popliteal Cyst) | Most knees with DJD have Baker's cysts. The cyst is not the problem, it is the result of the inflammation from the DJD. |
| Patellofemoral Pain (Runner's Knee) | Abnormal tracking of the knee cap leads to stress on the joint cartilage in that area. Ultimately this can lead to degeneration of the knee cap cartilage. |
| Rheumatoid/Inflammatory Arthritis | The cartilage of the knee is attacked or damaged by the disease state. As it gets damaged it triggers the secondary process of degeneration. |
| Anterior Cruciate Ligament (ACL) Tear | Many knees with DJD have ACL degeneration and/or tears. Healthy knees with ACL tears develop DJD at an accelerated rate. |

| | |
|---|---|
| Accidents, injuries, and fractures around the knee | Trauma to the joint surface can ultimately lead to degeneration. Fracture of the bones around the knee that change the alignment of the leg can lead to development of DJD at an accelerated rate. |
| Obesity and inactivity (poor muscle strength) | Excess force on the knee can lead to development of DJD at an accelerated rate, Weak muscles can't support the joint and can increase pain with DJD. Obesity increases force on the joint and can increase pain with DJD. |
| Malnutrition and dehydration | Creates a situation of unhealthy cartilage which can lead to development of DJD at an accelerated rate. |
| Depression/Anxiety | Although not a direct cause of DJD, these conditions have a direct impact on the amount and intensity of pain felt if DJD is present. Chronic knee pain may cause or trigger depression. |

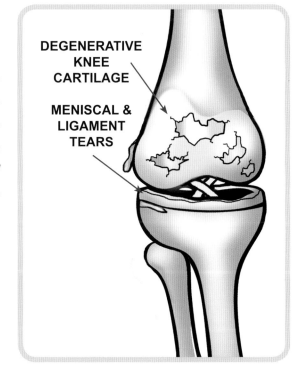

*Illustration shows a typical degenerative knee with wear of the joint cartilage, tears of the meniscus and degeneration of the ligaments.*

**DEGENERATIVE KNEE CARTILAGE**

**MENISCAL & LIGAMENT TEARS**

What all this means is that we should not focus too much or get hung up on the individual problems in the knee (eg. meniscal tears, Baker's cysts, etc.) and treating them with surgery initially. Of course, there are many cases where surgery does help, like an ACL tear in a young athlete (where reconstructing the ligament will help keep the knee more stable and avoid early degeneration) or replacing an end stage arthritic knee that has not responded to non-surgical treatments. However:

*"For most problems with the knee we should be focusing on making the knee as healthy as possible and doing our best to thwart degeneration of the knee."*

Now that may sound strange coming from me. I am, after all, an orthopedic surgeon, but I spend most of my day talking people *out of* surgery. That is, unless they have tried everything else (specifically what's in this book). "Everything else" – which actually works - involves lifestyle changes that are not drastic and may limit the need for medications, injections and invasive surgical procedures.

You might find this surprising, but surgery isn't the solution for many people who have a meniscus tear and arthritis in the knee severe enough to cause pain. A recent study published in *The New England Journal of Medicine* (one of medicine's most prestigious journals) showed that "most older people diagnosed with meniscus tears due to aging and arthritis get the same long-term relief with time and physical therapy as they do with surgery." [1] Studies have found similar results showing no benefit for treating osteoarthritis with arthroscopic surgery [2, 3]. Perhaps more concerning is that studies show that even the treatment for advanced arthritis, total knee replacement, leaves approximately 1 in 5 patients not satisfied with their outcome [4, 5, 6].

That said, knee surgery, when needed, can and does dramatically improve most people's lives. The good news is if surgery is needed, the foundation provided in this book will give the best chance of a successful outcome.

> "*Many of the patients that are unhappy after knee surgery have not put into place the appropriate measures to ensure a good result.*"

Let's now delve a bit more into the limitations of modern medicine.

Modern medicine has provided many benefits to mankind such as penicillin and the near eradication of polio, but when it comes to knees, as those studies I just told you about reinforce, less may be more. Why? Because what the doctor treats is more often the symptom rather than the cause.

One example is that surgery alone will not "fix" a bad knee if the patient is obese, sedentary and makes poor nutritional choices. Until those conditions change, healing and restoring knee health are severely impeded.

In addition, picture taking tools such as x-rays and MRIs aren't always worth a thousand words after all. At the very least they have no capacity to tell the whole story and can lead to "one size fits all" treatments.

Let me give you an example of the sort of limitation I'm talking about. X-rays or MRIs of two patients can show the same type and degree of arthritis in the knee – yet one of them plays tennis and golf three times a week and the other can't walk even a few steps to the mailbox without wincing in pain.

Why is that? Because the active person with the same apparent condition is most likely incorporating healthy practices into his lifestyle, and the other isn't. Surprisingly, the injury looks the same in the images of someone 100 pounds overweight as it does in a person of normal weight. The image is not telling the whole story. See where I'm going now when I talk about limitations?

Effective treatments, like those covered in this book, *do* take into account the whole story – the whole person – and look at factors such as the condition of the patient's muscles, their weight, their nutrition and their lifestyle.

Now, am I saying that you shouldn't get an x-ray or MRI? No, because these tools can be helpful at seeing what's wrong inside the knee, and occasionally there can be serious problems that need to be found.  However, for most routine cases of knee pain, they do not provide every piece of the puzzle – specifically the lifestyle pieces of that puzzle.

Oh, and one more thing. Remember what I said in Chapter 2: *Why* your knee is bad really doesn't matter much of the time. What does matter is how to make it feel better. And that's where non-invasive treatments come in, few of which have any bearing on what your doctor sees on your x-ray or MRI.

The next chapter will detail exactly what we're talking about, so turn the page and read on!

# 4

# THE COMPREHENSIVE SOLUTION: MAKING IT "ALL BETTER" WITH COMBINATION THERAPIES AND LIFESTYLE CHANGE

What you will learn in this chapter:

- Why I felt the need to do more for my patients than surgery alone

- What are "multi-modal therapy" and "lifestyle change" and why they can help

- The four components of a comprehensive approach: education, nutrition, fitness and support

- Bringing it all together into a lifestyle... A personal story

- Combining the four components achieves a "synergy," where the combined effects are greater than the individual components

If you've read this far you already know that even though I specialize in surgery, I only recommend it when people have tried everything to avoid it but have been unable to.

When I was a resident at Columbia University in New York City specializing in orthopedic surgery and later a Fellow at Harvard in reconstructive surgery of the hip and knee, I was there to learn the art of orthopedic surgery and joint replacement. Surgery was mostly what I thought about, studied and practiced. I did get to interact with some patients in the office and clinic setting, but didn't get to know them or really see how the surgical interventions I performed affected their lives. Nevertheless, learning to perform surgery was the highlight of my training.

Once I entered into private practice, however, and saw that although surgery helped the majority of people tremendously, many people with knee problems were not doing nearly as well after surgery as they had expected. I was forced to re-think my approach. Was there more I could be doing to help ensure a better result for my knee patients? I also saw that patients wanted to do everything they could to avoid having surgery. I asked myself, could I possibly help them postpone the need for surgery or even avoid surgery altogether?

I set my mind to find out.

*"Little by little I learned that knee health and knee surgery can be vastly affected both positively and negatively by lifestyle choices, as well as the patient's level of involvement in the management of their condition."*

I also realized that in many cases patients are actually more positively impacted when the surgeon keeps the scalpel tucked away (made possible when the patient adheres to a healthy lifestyle.) Over the years I have refined my system, incorporated all of the most important information available about knee health into it, and have made it the major focus of this book.

Patients often ask me, "What can I do to prevent my knee from hurting or from getting worse?" Others want to know how they can have the best possible outcome from surgery. Some, who have already had knee surgery and are still having some pain, want to know what can make them feel better. Well, the answer for many is to follow a system of "multi-modal" treatments and lifestyle change. Multi-modal is a fancy-sounding word that simply means a combination of actions you can take which work together to improve your chances of fixing your aching knee. Lifestyle change means putting in place the appropriate foundation to make your knees feel as good as possible despite anything that may be going on with them.

Before I get into the specifics, let's talk about what your knees have in common with your car: When you turn the key in the ignition, you expect it to start and drive smoothly. It usually does, as long as you have performed routine maintenance on it like changing the oil and rotating the tires. If you haven't…well, you're taking your chances.

The same holds true for your knees. Take care of them and they'll take care of you.

To help you do just that requires a four-part lifestyle program that you'll read about in more detail in subsequent chapters.

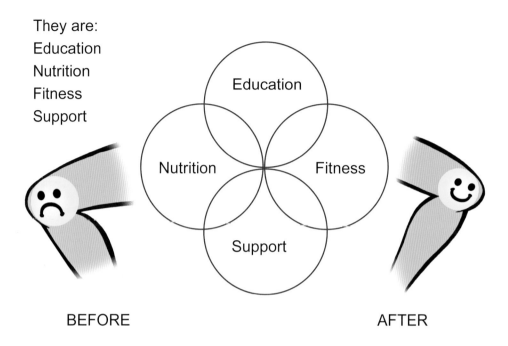

They are:
Education
Nutrition
Fitness
Support

BEFORE

AFTER

*Illustration shows the 4 components of a lifestyle program for creating healthy and happy knees.*

## EDUCATION

The more you know about your knee, your specific condition, pain control, lifestyle contributions and what you can expect from whatever treatment you decide upon, the better you can manage the outcome. Being educated also helps you communicate more clearly with your physician.

## NUTRITION

This chapter will detail the ways that being overweight can damage your knees and cause pain, and why losing just a few pounds can make a tremendous difference. We will discuss some simple ways to drop pounds and help unload your knees.

We'll discuss what foods you should and shouldn't eat to maximize your body's nutrition and minimize inflammation. Some foods can help minimize inflammation and make your knees happy. Certain processed foods, like white sugar and wheat, can cause inflammation making knees stiff and sore. Knowing what to avoid and what to eat will go a long way toward pain-free knees.

Some nutrients such as turmeric and glucosamine sulfate, have been shown in studies to reduce inflammation, decrease pain and promote health of the knee joint . Interestingly, some studies have indicated that these over-the-counter supplements may be just as effective as traditional medicine in relieving knee aches and pains.

## FITNESS

One of the best ways to keep your knees healthy and to help them heal, is to exercise regularly. Numerous studies confirm that exercise is the key to healthy and happy knees because it strengthens the muscles around the joint, increases flexibility and improves overall physical and mental fitness.

In the Fitness chapter we will tell you which exercises are best and provide you with a 10-minute program of exercises that are easy to do and easy to incorporate into your routine (no gym required!). Done regularly, your knees will get stronger and your chances of feeling better will vastly increase.

## SUPPORT

As our knees and bodies age, some occasional aches and pains are to be expected. It is important to know safe tricks and tips to manage these.

Support often helps when the pain starts interfering with your day (or is keeping you from exercising). When this occurs, there are some safe external remedies you can use.

Covered in the Support chapter are topical pain relief, compression and bracing.

Topical pain relievers will soothe sore knees. Compression garments can help the knee feel supported and reduce inflammation and swelling.

Utilizing over the counter drugs is also discussed.

## LIFESTYLE — BRINGING IT ALL TOGETHER

About 6 years ago my mother-in-law began complaining of pain in her knee that was not improving. Her well-being is vital to my family. Aside from being a loving mother and grandmother, she helps take care of my young children as well as prepares us delicious meals several times a week. Unfortunately, her x-rays revealed advanced osteoarthritis…….her knee was "bone on bone." Over time she had run through all the "conventional" treatments that medicine had to offer and was, quite frankly, headed toward knee replacement surgery. That is, until she implemented a lifestyle change. Now you can find her exercising at the YMCA each day or walking along the beach, taking a joint supplement, eating right, and using a topical pain reliever and knee support when needed. You can find her going up and down the stairs and playing with my kids. What you won't find her doing is complaining about her arthritic knee. Now I'm not saying that her knee is as good as when she was twenty and I'm not predicting she will never need knee replacement surgery (although it's looking good), but I do know her knee feels much better off now than it did six years ago. And I also know if she ever does need surgery, she has the foundation in place to have an excellent result.

Why was she able to feel better you ask? By combining these different methods to address a given problem, a synergy occurs. It is highly unlikely that she would have avoided surgery all these years had she just taken a supplement or just lost weight or just exercised. It was the combination of actions in her lifestyle which interacted to produce a bigger outcome than any one element could have done alone.

So now, turn the page, and let's take a closer look at the four components.

# 5

# EDUCATION

What you will learn in this chapter:

• Ignoring your knees won't help them improve

• Educating yourself about your knees enables you to take the steps necessary to improve the way your knees feel and function

• Every choice we make involves some risk, and we need to consider this

• Effectiveness of treatments varies, and can be hard to show in studies

• Part of educating yourself is understanding reasonable expectations for how your knees feel and function at different stages of life and doing everything possible to maximize how they perform

• How learning about the significant impact of weight loss on knee health resulted in a patient avoiding surgery

Renowned British author Aldous Huxley wrote in his Complete Essays that "Facts do not cease to exist because they are ignored."

It's true for many things, and knee health is certainly one of them.

Ignoring knee pain or taking a passive approach to your condition is highly unlikely to result in any improvement.

*"Just as being aware of your surroundings can help keep you safe, conscious awareness of your knees can greatly improve the chances you will protect them."*

By reading this book you're already taking the giant step of educating yourself in several ways:

You are learning about the parts of the knee and how those parts can go wrong. But more importantly, you are learning about why pain in the knee occurs and what you can do to make your knees feel as good as possible, despite what may be going on inside the knee.

You are learning about nutrition - which foods are detrimental to your knee health and which foods and supplements are advantageous to it, promoting more consciousness about what you are putting in your body.

You are learning that exercise in general, and strengthening the muscles around the knee are vital to the long term health of the knee.

You are learning about what medicine and surgery have to offer when your knee hurts, and some things that should be tried before resorting to those riskier options. The information will help you achieve the best possible outcome should surgery be required.

Being armed with knowledge will also help you communicate better with your doctor. Becoming an active partner with your physician when medical intervention is appropriate can have a significant impact on a desirable outcome.

As we select treatments for our knees, there are three critical concepts to understand. The first is risk, the second is effectiveness, and the third is expectations.

## RISK

Pretty much every decision we make in life has some potential risk. Risk is defined as the potential loss or undesired consequence resulting from an intervention or lack of intervention. When we drive our cars we risk death, but we don't think about it a lot because we need to utilize cars to get where we need to go and lead a productive life. But, imagine if there were a warning label you had to review prior to getting in your car of all the terrible things that could happen to you if an accident were to occur. I imagine you would be quite concerned, and maybe even scared to drive. Medical treatments are no different, but we think about them a lot more because we don't utilize them every day…….that is until we need to.

Treatments for the knee specifically vary from the least risky (lifestyle modifications), intermediate (medications and injections), to the most risky (surgical intervention). Sometimes I encounter patients that for whatever reason, wish to rush right to surgery without trying some of the most basic and safer things. They feel their knee is broken and must be fixed. This is foolish! I tell all my patients that every day in life is precious and you never know what the future holds, so never take more risk in life than is necessary at that time. When less risky things are tried and are not sufficient, everyone can feel more comfortable moving forward with taking more risk, and therefore be more willing to deal with whatever the outcome may be. There are no guarantees that any treatment will work or be entirely safe. With all that said, when you have a knee problem, there is also risk to doing nothing. If you ignore the problem altogether it may worsen. Chronic pain and stiffness can develop leading to inactivity, depression, weight gain........all counterproductive. The most important thing is to be honest with yourself about how your knee condition affects your quality of life and intervene when needed taking into consideration the risk of the treatments versus their effectiveness.

## EFFECTIVENESS

Effectiveness is defined as the ability of something to be successful in producing a desired result. Ideally, the best treatments for any problem would be highly effective, with little risk involved. Unfortunately, there is no magic treatment that works for everyone and there is no treatment that is safe for everyone. Complicating matters further, it is difficult to determine effectiveness. Medical studies are commonly inconclusive or have contradictory results to prior studies on the topic. In fact, one recent study published in the Mayo Clinic Proceedings found that when a study is undertaken to test the so called "standard of care" (the recognized treatment for a condition), the results of the study are just as likely to disprove that treatment as to reaffirm it [7]. This does not necessarily suggest that these treatments don't work, it's just that it can be hard to prove in studies.

So if doctors and scientists have trouble determining which treatments are effective, how does an individual patient with no medical background figure out what will work for them?  This brings us back to our above discussion about risk.

*"Start first with the things that are currently known or thought to work, that don't involve much risk. Only go to riskier treatments if the safer alternatives are not effective."*

## EXPECTATIONS

A big part of determining whether or not a treatment is effective has to do with the concept of expectations.  With or without problems or treatments, there is a big difference in what we can expect from our knees when we are 20 years old, versus 50 years old, versus 80 years old.  At 20 years old, our knees typically are in the ideal state of health. The cartilage and meniscus are thick and well lubricated.  The muscles, tendons, and ligaments are healthy and strong.  In this state, usually we don't even notice or think about our knees, because they are working perfectly. Treatments at this stage should have the goal of restoring the knee back to this state of well being and can be judged accordingly.  At around 50 years old, the cartilage typically has some degree of wear (you can't expect there to be no wear on your car tires after driving around for 50,000 miles……..and our knees are no different.) Occasional aches and pains can be common, particularly with high intensity or prolonged activity.  The goal of any treatment at this stage of life should be to manage and minimize these aches and pains.  By 80 years old, many of our knees are seriously worn out. Pain and stiffness can be frequent. Many people by this age will have already had or be considering knee replacement surgery. The goal at this stage of life is to minimize pain and preserve function and mobility. The goal should not be unachievable, like having a knee that feels as good as when you were 20 years old. The most important thing to understand is the need to put in place the foundation to maximize the way our knees function and feel, regardless of the stage of life or what they have been through.

## THE POWER OF EDUCATION

The following anecdote illustrates the power of knowledge and the undeniable benefit of good doctor-patient communication.

A 55-year-old schoolteacher came to see me one September with extremely damaged knees due, in large part, to the fact that she was about 70 pounds overweight and wasn't exercising. She had been told by another physician that she needed surgery, and I agreed that if nothing changed, that was her only option. The first time she had available for the procedure was winter break, so we scheduled it for December. During that initial appointment I educated her about the benefits to her knees of losing weight and exercise, which she obviously took to heart, because when she came back to my office a week before her surgery date, she had lost 40 pounds and was stronger. Her knees were feeling so much better that we were able to cancel her operation. Had she not been educated about the dramatic benefit of weight loss to the knees, she would have spent the holidays recovering from surgery instead of celebrating with friends and family.

So, now that you know why becoming educated is so important, let's delve a little deeper into what you need to know.

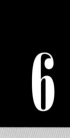

# NUTRITION

What you will learn in this chapter:

- For every pound your body carries around, your knees endure four pounds of pressure

- Losing a small amount of weight greatly magnifies the relief to the pressure on your knees

- Obesity is a major factor in osteoarthritis because of increased pressure on the joints and changes in body composition

- The "low fat" diet craze of the 80s started America on a path of obesity in numbers never seen before, followed by the "low carb" craze

- Artificial sweeteners are making Americans fatter, not thinner

- Cutting portion sizes can help you lose weight while still eating the things you love

- One of the biggest advantages of managing pain and inflammation with nutrition is not exposing yourself to the possible adverse side effects of prescription medications

- At least 80 percent of the American diet is made up of foods that promote inflammation

- A diet similar to the "Mediterranean diet" can help to significantly reduce inflammation. This involves cutting out certain foods like white flour while emphasizing plenty of fruits and vegetables

- Water is an important component of a healthy diet

- Smoking tobacco has been linked to knee pain and cartilage loss

- Certain nutritional supplements may help reduce pain and inflammation. These include glucosamine sulfate and turmeric, which are time tested and safe for most adults

When it comes to our knees, there are 4 important aspects regarding nutrition that are important to understand including:

1. Weight Management
2. Knowing what to eat and drink
3. Knowing what to avoid or limit eating and drinking
4. The role of supplements

## Weight Management

Did you know that for each pound your body carries around, your knees endure four pounds of pressure? That means if you weigh 200 pounds, there are 800 pounds exerted on your knees every time you walk. And that's just for someone who's engaged in normal day-to-day activity. If you do more, such as climbing stairs or high impact exercise like tennis or jogging, the pressure is even greater.

On the flip side of the mathematical equation, losing even a small amount of weight magnifies the benefit.

*"A ten-pound loss relieves 40 pounds*
*of pressure on your knees"*

Imagine carrying around a five gallon jug of water (about 40 pounds) and then letting it down….how much better would that feel?

With so many people overweight in this country it's no wonder there are millions of people limping around with bad knees and why we have the highest percentage of knee replacement surgeries performed in the world. Just how many people are overweight? According to the Centers for Disease Control, an astonishing 70 percent of adults in the U.S. are overweight, and that includes the 35 percent who are considered obese (in Japan, only about 3 percent of people are obese). In 2013, the American Medical Association classified obesity as a disease.

Obesity is defined as a Body Mass Index (BMI) of 30 or higher. The height and weight of the individual are used to calculate BMI. It classifies people as underweight, normal, overweight, and obese. It may be an inaccurate tool in people who are in exceptionally good shape (not too many of those people out there!) Use the table to measure yours.

## BODY MASS INDEX (BMI) CHART FOR ADULTS

Categories: Underweight | Healthy | Overweight | Obese | Extremely Obese

| Weight lbs | 100 | 105 | 110 | 115 | 120 | 125 | 130 | 135 | 140 | 145 | 150 | 155 | 160 | 165 | 170 | 175 | 180 | 185 | 190 | 195 | 200 | 205 | 210 | 215 |
|---|---|---|---|---|---|---|---|---|---|---|---|---|---|---|---|---|---|---|---|---|---|---|---|---|
| **Kgs** | 45.5 | 47.7 | 50.0 | 52.3 | 54.5 | 56.8 | 59.1 | 61.4 | 63.6 | 65.9 | 68.2 | 70.5 | 72.7 | 75.0 | 77.3 | 79.5 | 81.8 | 84.1 | 86.4 | 88.6 | 90.9 | 93.2 | 95.5 | 97.7 |
| **Height in/cm** | | | | | | | | | | | | | | | | | | | | | | | | |
| 5'00" - 152.4 | 19 | 20 | 21 | 22 | 23 | 24 | 25 | 26 | 27 | 28 | 29 | 30 | 31 | 32 | 33 | 34 | 35 | 36 | 37 | 38 | 39 | 40 | 41 | 42 |
| 5'01" - 154.9 | 18 | 19 | 20 | 21 | 22 | 23 | 24 | 25 | 26 | 27 | 28 | 29 | 30 | 31 | 32 | 33 | 34 | 35 | 36 | 36 | 37 | 38 | 39 | 40 |
| 5'02" - 157.4 | 18 | 19 | 20 | 21 | 22 | 22 | 23 | 24 | 25 | 26 | 27 | 28 | 29 | 30 | 31 | 32 | 33 | 33 | 34 | 35 | 36 | 37 | 38 | 39 |
| 5'03" - 160.0 | 17 | 18 | 19 | 20 | 21 | 22 | 23 | 24 | 24 | 25 | 26 | 27 | 28 | 29 | 30 | 31 | 32 | 32 | 33 | 34 | 35 | 36 | 37 | 38 |
| 5'04" - 162.5 | 17 | 18 | 18 | 19 | 20 | 21 | 22 | 23 | 24 | 24 | 25 | 26 | 27 | 28 | 29 | 30 | 31 | 31 | 32 | 33 | 34 | 35 | 36 | 37 |
| 5'05" - 165.1 | 16 | 17 | 18 | 19 | 20 | 20 | 21 | 22 | 23 | 24 | 25 | 25 | 26 | 27 | 28 | 29 | 30 | 30 | 31 | 32 | 33 | 34 | 35 | 35 |
| 5'06" - 167.6 | 16 | 17 | 17 | 18 | 19 | 20 | 21 | 21 | 22 | 23 | 24 | 25 | 25 | 26 | 27 | 28 | 29 | 29 | 30 | 31 | 32 | 33 | 34 | 34 |
| 5'07" - 170.1 | 15 | 16 | 17 | 18 | 18 | 19 | 20 | 21 | 22 | 22 | 23 | 24 | 25 | 25 | 26 | 27 | 28 | 29 | 29 | 30 | 31 | 32 | 33 | 33 |
| 5'08" - 172.7 | 15 | 16 | 16 | 17 | 18 | 19 | 19 | 20 | 21 | 22 | 22 | 23 | 24 | 25 | 25 | 26 | 27 | 28 | 28 | 29 | 30 | 31 | 32 | 32 |
| 5'09" - 175.2 | 14 | 15 | 16 | 17 | 17 | 18 | 19 | 20 | 20 | 21 | 22 | 22 | 23 | 24 | 25 | 25 | 26 | 27 | 28 | 28 | 29 | 30 | 31 | 31 |
| 5'10" - 177.8 | 14 | 15 | 15 | 16 | 17 | 18 | 18 | 19 | 20 | 20 | 21 | 22 | 22 | 23 | 24 | 25 | 25 | 26 | 27 | 28 | 28 | 29 | 30 | 30 |
| 5'11" - 180.3 | 14 | 14 | 15 | 16 | 16 | 17 | 18 | 18 | 19 | 20 | 21 | 31 | 22 | 23 | 23 | 24 | 25 | 25 | 26 | 27 | 27 | 28 | 29 | 30 |
| 6'00" - 182.8 | 13 | 14 | 14 | 15 | 16 | 17 | 17 | 18 | 19 | 19 | 20 | 21 | 21 | 22 | 23 | 23 | 24 | 25 | 25 | 26 | 27 | 27 | 28 | 29 |
| 6'01" - 185.4 | 13 | 13 | 14 | 15 | 15 | 16 | 17 | 17 | 18 | 19 | 19 | 20 | 21 | 21 | 22 | 23 | 23 | 24 | 25 | 25 | 26 | 27 | 27 | 28 |
| 6'02" - 187.9 | 12 | 13 | 14 | 14 | 15 | 16 | 16 | 17 | 18 | 18 | 19 | 19 | 20 | 21 | 21 | 22 | 23 | 23 | 24 | 25 | 25 | 26 | 27 | 27 |
| 6'03" - 190.5 | 12 | 13 | 13 | 14 | 15 | 15 | 16 | 16 | 17 | 18 | 18 | 19 | 20 | 20 | 21 | 21 | 22 | 23 | 23 | 24 | 25 | 25 | 26 | 26 |
| 6'04" - 193.0 | 12 | 12 | 13 | 14 | 14 | 15 | 15 | 16 | 17 | 17 | 18 | 18 | 19 | 20 | 20 | 21 | 22 | 22 | 23 | 23 | 24 | 25 | 25 | 26 |

Obesity and knee osteoarthritis go hand-in-hand due to increased pressure on the joint and changes in body composition. In fact, studies have shown that people who are obese are four times more likely to have osteoarthritis in their knees than the general population [8].

*"Two in three people who are obese may develop symptomatic knee OA in their lifetime [9]."*

Therefore, getting rid of excess weight is a crucial component of good knee health. The benefit of weight loss is demonstrated in the example below:

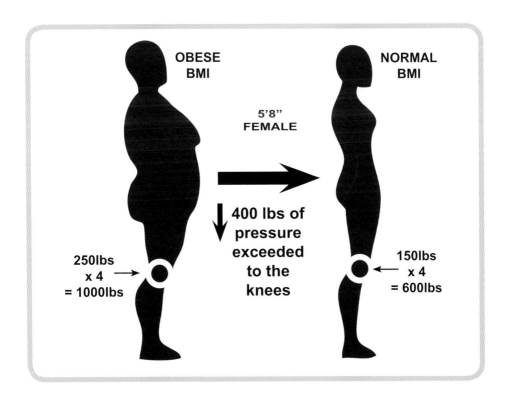

**First a little background:**

Many factors have contributed to the fattening of America, but one of the biggest culprits is the food industry, which responded in the late 1980s to reports that the American diet included too much saturated fat. To meet consumers' demands for products with less saturated fat, they came out with products made instead with unsaturated vegetable oil (which has as many calories as any other form of fat) or they significantly reduced the fat content of the foods. To make lower-fat concoctions tasty, they added sugar and other fat-promoting carbohydrates for flavor.

Consumers saw the "low fat" or "no saturated fat" labels and were lulled into thinking these foods were good for them and OK to eat (and maybe ate more of). In fact, these foods frequently had just as many calories as their predecessors and now contained ingredients which contributed to weight gain.

The same phenomenon has occurred more recently with the low-carb craze. Remember that just because a food item is low-carb doesn't mean it's healthy for you. Those foods can still be very high in calories, contain little nutrition and have ingredients that promote weight gain.

Another potential contributor to America's obesity problem is the proliferation of artificial sweeteners, especially in soft drinks. Now, you'd think these would be better for your waistline, but an analysis of a dozen studies on diet drinks showed the opposite [10].

The researchers found that just as with regular soda, artificially sweetened beverages are associated with obesity, type 2 diabetes, metabolic syndrome and cardiovascular disease. It may also cause disruption of the metabolism.

## WHAT TO DO:

My advice? It's all about portion control. You can eat pretty much anything you want in appropriate portions........which are probably way smaller than you think they should be. I recommend avoiding processed foods as much as possible. Stick with whole foods like fish, chicken, vegetables and whole grains and turn to foods like fruits and nuts for snacking. Drink water and unsweetened beverages. Avoid fad diets which are not sustainable.

One of the most common things I hear from my patients is "Doc, I can't lose weight because I can't exercise. I'm in too much pain." However, this is not the reason why people can't lose weight because exercise is a surprisingly minor component of the weight loss puzzle. You can spend a half hour on a treadmill and burn just 250 calories – easily negated by eating one cookie. It's almost all about how much and what you put in your body.

Now don't misunderstand me. Exercise is absolutely essential to good knee health (and good overall health, too). It can provide a "supporting" role for weight loss. The main benefit, however, is not its impact on weight loss but rather its significant bearing on cardiovascular health, muscle strength, flexibility, and mental well being.

So, let's turn our attention to diet (and by this I don't mean "a diet," I mean what you choose every day of your life to put in your mouth as part of your healthy lifestyle). Let's start by talking about my diet.

In the summer of 2012 I vacationed with my family in Europe. I am 30-pounds lighter today than I was then because of what I observed there.

The Europeans didn't seem to be "dieting." Everyone was eating what they wanted – pasta, sauces, meat, desserts. The difference? The portions were considerably smaller than what is typical in America.

My observation inspired me to start cutting my portion sizes by half what I would normally eat to see what happened. If I normally would eat a sandwich for lunch, I started to give the other half away. If I normally had two slices of pizza, I started to eat only one. I called this my "half portion diet," because I essentially took what I used to eat and started to eat half that amount. I also added a glass of water before each meal, followed by a glass of water afterwards, and a small treat such as a piece of dark chocolate to finish it off and signify the end of the meal. After the meal, I immediately would move on with my day or night and no longer think about food until the next meal.

### THE HALF PORTION DIET
### A 4-STEP PLAN TO LOSING WEIGHT

1. Drink a glass of water before and after each meal
2. Eat half portions of what you normally would eat
3. Finish with a small amount of something sweet
4. Distract yourself ... move on with your day or evening

Much to my surprise, not only did the weight come off but within a few minutes I felt completely satisfied, even though I had eaten less.

*" I learned that when you are inclined to, say, get a second helping, if you wait just a few minutes you won't want it anymore."*

As I started to see the benefits of losing weight and feeling better about myself, I started to take a closer look at what and how I was eating. I was in the habit of skipping breakfast, grabbing some sort of unhealthy snack for lunch at the office and then binging at dinner because I was so famished.

Today I eat four regularly spaced out meals a day (breakfast, lunch, afternoon snack and dinner). One example of an afternoon "meal" is a snack of an apple and 5 to 10 almonds. I never skip meals! I also started making smarter food choices, avoiding processed foods such as white bread  and making better choices like broccoli dipped into hummus rather than a bag of chips (which satisfies the urge for something crunchy). I drink only water and unsweetened beverages (water with lemon, lime or a spash of fruit juice, iced tea or iced coffee, etc).

Those are some of the tips and tricks I use to lose weight and keep my weight down, and here are ten more tips I particularly like:

• Learn appropriate portion sizes. Put more vegetables on your plate than meat or starch.  Half your plate should be vegetables, one quarter protein (lean meat, eggs, fish etc.) and one quarter carbohydrates (rice, pasta , bread, etc).

• Weigh yourself at least once a week, if your weight is not decreasing then you are still eating too much. Cut your portions further and weigh in the next week.

• Plan your meals ahead of time and don't skip meals. A thought-out meal is likely to be much healthier than an impulsive one.

- Avoid processed foods as much as possible. Stick to whole foods.
- Use smaller plates. The larger the plate the more you will serve yourself.
- Slow down when you eat. The faster you eat, the more you eat.
- Don't deprive yourself of the foods you love, like pasta or ice cream. Just eat them less often and in a smaller amount.
- Be very cautious eating out at restaurants. Cut all food in half and take home or share the other portion.
- Put healthy foods like fruit out on the counter where you can see them and grab them easily.
- Get enough sleep. When you're sleep deprived you are likely to make all sorts of poor choices, including choices about what you eat.

The most important thing to know is that ANYONE can lose weight. I realize that many people have been heavy their whole lives, some people have thyroid issues, some people are diabetic, and that it can be difficult to exercise with bad knees. Regardless, if the proper habits are established it is quite possible to get your extra weight off and feel better than you have ever felt! Try the half portion diet as described and you are likely to see success as I did.

## DIET

One of the biggest advantages of managing pain and inflammation with nutrition is that you are not exposing yourself to the possible adverse side effects of prescription medications. It almost always makes sense to go the nutritional route first.

Now, there's a lot of information available all over the place about good nutrition, so what I want to talk about in this book is nutrition explicit to knee and joint health, specifically foods that reduce (or trigger) inflammation.

*"Joint pain is often caused by inflammation, and inflammation is caused to a large degree by what we eat."*

It's estimated that at least 80 percent of the American diet is made up of foods that promote inflammation. These include: refined sugar/grains/cooking oils/flour, full-fat dairy products, many fast foods and fatty red meat.

If your knees are hurting, you may want to consider getting those inflammatory foods out of your diet as much as possible, especially if the cause of that pain is related to arthritis.

An anti-inflammatory diet is often compared to the "Mediterranean diet." It's comprised primarily of fruits, vegetables, raw nuts and healthy proteins such as lean meat, fish and fish oil supplements, walnuts, eggs and skinless poultry. It can also include whole grains like brown rice and bulgur wheat. A little red wine is OK, and so is dark chocolate (one of my favorites). Choose olive oil or coconut oil instead of refined cooking oils, and always choose real butter over margarine.

Besides being good for you, anti-inflammatory foods don't have to be bland, because some wonderful spices have anti-inflammatory benefits. These include ginger, curry, rosemary, oregano, garlic, coriander and turmeric (more about turmeric in a moment). Use them creatively and plentifully.

*"Drinking water is also an important part
of a diet for healthy knees."*

Many people in America are walking around somewhat dehydrated. We all know that we are supposed to drink 8 glasses of water a day (at least), but how many of us actually do it? We now know that most of our joint cartilage is made of water and that water is a critical component of knee health. By drinking a glass of water before and after each meal, you can ensure proper hydration and also help fill your belly so you don't overeat.

One other important thing is if you are a smoker, then you should quit if you want to have healthy knees. Smoking has been linked to increased knee pain and progression of cartilage loss [11]. Even worse, if you are a smoker and then require surgery, your chances of having a serious complication increase significantly [12, 13].

## SUPPLEMENTS

Let's talk now about supplements which are sometimes called nutraceuticals.

Enter a health food store or open up a health magazine and you find yourself in a very confusing world. Each product touts amazing benefits, or at least implies them. This is because the Food and Drug Administration does not regulate these substances because they are not considered drugs. So what's a person to do who just wants their knee to feel better?

While some supplements have very little basis for the claims made about them, there are some that have been tried by people all over the world and have been shown to work in numerous studies. Those are the ones I am going to tell you about because I believe in them. I've seen many of my patients improve who have used them. Now certainly supplements are controversial, and even the most popular ones have studies that support their use and studies that conclude that they don't help (remember our discussion on effectiveness and how unreliable studies can be from Chapter 5). However, if you poll patients, many find them extremely helpful. Many doctors, including myself, continue to recommend supplements believed to be safe and effective for most patients despite the powers that be telling us we should not. Why? Because they are, in general, much safer than a lot of the other treatments out there and are worth a trial. Nothing works for everyone, so you start with the least risky options first.

## GLUCOSAMINE SULFATE:

So what is glucosamine sulfate? It's a natural substance produced by the body and found in cartilage and joint fluid. It is arguably one of the most studied "natural remedies" in existence.

According to the Mayo Clinic there is "good evidence to support the use of glucosamine sulfate in the treatment of mild-to-moderate knee osteoarthritis" [14]. In addition, the National Institutes of Health (NIH) lists glucosamine sulfate as "likely effective" for osteoarthritis [15]. However some recent reviews and guidelines have concluded the opposite. The truth probably lies somewhere in between. Again, nothing works for everyone. However there have been so many studies that show beneficial effects of glucosamine, particularly for knees, and it is widely thought to be safe for almost everyone (more on this below).

So why are there many studies that say glucosamine doesn't

work? There are several reasons. First, there are different types. Many of the studies that showed glucosamine was effective utilized glucosamine sulfate in an appropriate dose of 1500 mg daily. However, many studies use a different substance called glucosamine hydrochloride (much more commonly available in the United States and according to NIH is rated as "insufficient evidence" for osteoarthritis and knee pain) and so the results may not be comparable to glucosamine sulfate. Second, many studies mix the glucosamine with chondroitin sulfate which may not be beneficial and may ultimately lower the dose of glucosamine needed or the effectiveness of glucosamine. Third, some of the studies that found glucosamine similar to a placebo also found that the traditional medications used to treat arthritis (these are called NSAID's) were also no different than a placebo. So it is quite possible it is the lack of our ability to prove effectiveness that is part of the problem. Making matters even more confusing, is that many researchers and physicians that are performing or evaluating these studies are supported financially by the traditional pharmaceutical industry, creating a potential for bias against natural treatments.

While the debate goes on, glucosamine continues to be the most widely utilized supplement for joints and Americans currently spend close to 1 billion dollars on glucosamine supplements annually. People continue to vote with their wallets. It remains widely utilized in veterinary medicine, where it has for decades, been believed to help animals with their pain and function.

It's not known for sure what glucosamine sulfate does or how it works, but it is fairly clear it does not regrow cartilage that has been lost. The debate really is about relief or avoidance of symptoms (pain, stiffness, function, etc) and the ability of glucosamine sulfate to protect the joint from damage.

Glucosamine is not a treatment for the impatient. It takes eight to twelve weeks, possibly even longer, for the benefits of glucosamine to be noticeable. Some people will benefit more than others.

Occasionally my patients taking glucosamine tell me they think they notice improvements but they aren't sure. If they've been on it for at least three months, I advise them to stop taking it for a couple of weeks and see how they feel. If they start experiencing more pain, they know it's helping. You can try this, too.

According to the NIH, glucosamine sulfate is considered "likely safe" when used appropriately by adults. It should not be taken during pregnancy or while breast feeding. People with asthma should be cautious using it, as there may be a linkage. It is generally safe for most people with diabetes, but blood sugar should be closely monitored. Although there are no reports of reactions, since most formulations are made from shells, people with shellfish allergies should be cautious. Like many natural treatments, glucosamine can interact with warfarin (Coumadin) causing the blood to be excessively thin. Thus its use should be avoided or closely monitored by a physician in patients taking strong blood thinners.

## TURMERIC

Turmeric is a spice used in Indian and Asian cuisine that has been shown to possess anti-inflammatory properties. It comes from the root of the Curcuma longa plant. Its orange and yellow pigment is called curcumin, which is believed to be the primary pharmacologic agent in turmeric.

Tumeric, in addition to being one of the most studied "natural remedies", has been utilized for thousands of years for medicinal purposes. The NIH now lists turmeric as "possibly effective" for osteoarthritis and notes that "some research shows that taking some turmeric extracts can reduce the pain caused by osteoarthritis of the knee."

A study published in 2009 compared curcumin with ibuprofen and reported that curcumin eased pain and improved function as well as ibuprofen (eg. motrin, advil) [17]. Other studies have found curcumin to be comparable in effectiveness to diclofenac (voltaren) [18] and celecoxib (Celebrex)[19].

The mechanism by which turmeric appears to work is by inhibiting some of the enzymes in the body thought to be responsible for inflammation, similar to the way traditional NSAIDS work [20]. Another way turmeric may help knees is by potentially avoiding depression (which we have already discussed has a link to chronic knee pain.) A recent study has demonstrated that turmeric can be as effective for treating depression as fluoexitine (prozac), a commonly prescribed anti-depressant drug [21].

Turmeric is considered "likely safe" by the NIH. It may have some blood thinning properties and should be avoided prior to surgery. It can interact with certain over-the-counter and prescription medications. If you're taking Coumadin, Plavix or aspirin, it can affect your blood's ability to clot and increase risk of bleeding. There also is some evidence that people with gall bladder issues should avoid taking tumeric.

By losing weight if needed and by maintaining an appropriate body weight, we can minimize the stress on our knees. Knowing what to eat and drink, what to avoid and which are the best supplements that we know of at this time can allow your knees to feel and function as good as possible.

Next we will discuss the important effects of exercise on your knees.

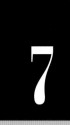

# FITNESS

What you will learn in this chapter:

- Regular exercise is one of the best ways to keep knees healthy and help painful knees improve

- Exercise is important, even if doing it hurts a little (but if it hurts a lot, stop!)

- Studies have shown that people who consistently do low-impact exercise and strength training have less pain and improved mobility

- Doing some kind of exercise is always better than doing nothing at all

- Exercise at least five days a week

- Stretching is important for maintaining flexibility

- Exercise doesn't have to be done all at once. Spread it throughout the day. Look for opportunities to exercise, like taking the stairs instead of the elevator

- Vary your exercise so you work different muscle groups

- Regular exercise leads to a state of physical and mental fitness

- Maximize your level of fitness before having knee surgery, as the condition you are in before you have it impacts the outcome

If I told you there was an extremely safe "natural" drug that you could take that would alleviate your knee pain, increase your mobility, fight depression and anxiety, help you lose weight and improve almost all aspects of your health, you would most certainly want to take it. Imagine further that this drug was free of cost, so everyone could have access to it. Amazingly, this drug exists and it is called exercise. Unfortunately, in America only about 1 in 5 people get the recommended level of physical activity.

> *"One of the best ways to keep your knees healthy, and to help them heal when they aren't, is regular exercise."*

Now maybe your reaction is: "But Dr. Martin, I can't exercise. It hurts too much! I feel like the Tin Man from the Wizard of Oz every day when I get out of bed." And I hear what you're saying, but stick with me here…

Study after study confirms that exercise is the key to strong, healthy knees – even knees that hurt when they move.

One published review of 197 studies conducted between 1970 and 2012 that examined nonsurgical and non-drug treatments for osteoarthritis-related knee pain concluded that *people with knee pain benefited from exercise* [22]. There was evidence that aerobic exercise and strength training reduced pain and improved the ease of getting around.

The key for folks getting the most from that kind of exercise, as well as for those doing other types, was commitment. Those who stayed with the program benefitted the most.

Exercise builds endurance, allowing us to walk longer distances without getting fatigued.

Exercise strengthens the muscles around the joint. The stronger the muscles, the more support they give the joint. The more support they give, the less likely your knees are to hurt. Strong muscles also help us balance and avoid falls.

Exercise also increases flexibility, making movement easier and reducing stiffness.

Exercise can also help with relaxation and mental health, limiting the influence of depression and anxiety on how your knees feel. Studies have found that exercise can be just as effective as taking anti-depressant drugs [23].

When the combination of all the above factors exist a state of "fitness" is achieved.

**There are 4 components of a balanced fitness program for the knee. These include:**

1. Endurance/Cardiovascular/General Health
   *Eg. walking, biking, elliptical trainers, stationary bike, recumbent bike*
2. Strength and Balance
   *Eg. 10 minute program below*
3. Stretching and Flexibility
   *Eg. quad, hamstring and hip stretches, yoga*
4. Cool down and Relaxation
   *Eg. tai-chi, meditation*

One of the most difficult things about exercise is making up your mind that you're going to do it, then actually doing it. Remember, a journey of 1,000 miles begins with a single step. I recommend starting out gently and always check with your physician prior to starting any new exercise program.

When it comes to exercise, doing something is always better than doing nothing. And there is always something you can do. It's important that you enjoy what you do, or otherwise you won't do it. If you don't like one type of exercise, try another, and keep looking. It might be a stationary bike, swimming or walking. It could be an elliptical trainer or a recumbent bicycle. Maybe you'll enjoy taking a bike ride after breakfast or a brisk walk after dinner each night. Another key is incorporating music that you enjoy, because it helps motivate you. It's also good to exercise with a spouse or friend. Using the "buddy system" reduces the chances that you'll cancel.

Once you've found a mode of exercise that you enjoy, incorporate it into your schedule for at least 30 minutes per day, no fewer than five days a week. To minimize discomfort, start your routine with some warm-up exercises. Stretching is good for maintaining motion and flexibility.

No time you say? Well, you can always find time for what is important (would you spend time chatting on the phone with an old friend who called whom you haven't heard from in years?). Believe me when I tell you, keeping your knees healthy is important if you want to stay off the sidelines of life.

Find ways to exercise when you're at home and when you're on vacation. You don't need a gym or fancy equipment. Just use the force and resistance of your body.

It doesn't have to be done all at once. Try ten minutes of stretching when you wake up. Take a 20 minute walk after dinner. Look for ways to "sneak" exercise into your routine, like using the stairs at work instead of the elevator or choosing a parking spot further away from the mall.

Be aware of this:

> *"If what you're doing doesn't aggravate your condition, it is helping it!"*

It's important to vary your exercise routine so that you work different muscle groups. Walk one day, swim the next. Variation makes exercising both more challenging and more interesting.

Don't worry if you feel a little muscular soreness or joint discomfort afterwards. Even when I was 20 years old and in great shape and worked out, I would feel sore the next day. A little discomfort is a small price to pay for strengthening your muscles, improving your flexibility (and helping your heart, too). It's normal to experience some achiness after exercising, particularly if you are out of shape.

If your knee is sore the next day, lay a towel over it and place an ice pack on the area for about 10-20 minutes. See chapter 8 for more on what to do when it hurts.

With everything I've said above, I must add one word of caution. Avoid any exercise that causes significant pain. I'm not a big fan of frequent or excessive, repetitive high impact exercises for people older than 30 or for anyone with an alignment issue (bowlegged or knock kneed). Examples of high impact exercises are running and jumping. Like most things, these are OK in moderation, but if you're running several miles a day, 7 days a week, you can expect that to eventually catch up with you.

Now, what about the person who is going to have surgery? If that's you, you probably think you get a pass here, since the procedure is designed to make you "good as new." Well, think again.

*"The kind of shape you're in before the operation has a big impact on how well you do afterwards."*

The stronger and more flexible you are before the surgery, the more likely you are to have a good outcome. So get going!

Below is a simple, effective exercise program that I encourage the knee patients in my practice to do for improved strength, flexibility and mobility. It can be done in ten minutes a day. This program was designed by the greatest physical therapist I know, Bob Habib, RPT. These exercises help my patients, and I know they will help you, too.

**ALWAYS CHECK WITH YOUR PHYSICIAN PRIOR TO STARTING ANY NEW EXERCISE ROUTINE.**

EACH EXERCISE SHOULD BE PERFORMED 20 TIMES WITH EACH LEG.

TAKE 3 DEEP BREATHS BETWEEN EACH EXERCISE SET. DURING THE EXERCISES DON'T FORGET TO BREATHE (IN THROUGH YOUR NOSE, AND OUT THROUGH YOUR MOUTH AS YOU EXERT YOURSELF).

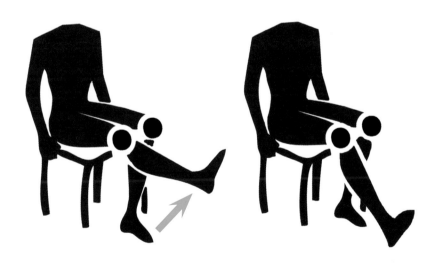

## SEATED LONG ARC QUAD - LAQ
Sit up straight in a chair, both feet flat on the floor, tighten your abdomen. Extend one leg in front of you, with your toes pointing

upward. Make sure your knee is fully extended (straight). Don't raise your thigh off the chair. Hold for 3 to 5 seconds then lower your leg slowly. Switch and repeat with the other leg.

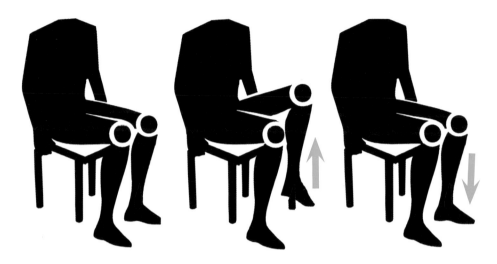

## SEATED MARCHING

Sit up straight in a chair, both feet flat on the floor with your arms crossed. Draw up one knee toward your chest, your toes pointed up the entire time. Set it down slowly back to the original position and then alternate to your other side. Make sure that the movement is rhythmic .

## HIP ABDUCTION - SINGLE- SEATED - STRAIGHT LEG

Start by sitting close to the edge of a chair with your target leg straight at the knee. Next, slide your target leg to the side. You can slide your heel across the floor. Then return to straight ahead. Keep your toes pointed up the entire time.

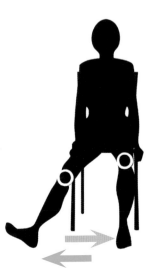

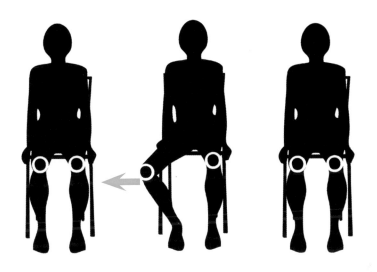

## HIP ABDUCTION - SINGLE- SEATED

Start by sitting close to the edge of a chair with knees bent and both feet on the floor. Next, move your target knee out to the side as shown and then return to straight ahead. Keep your feet on the floor the entire time.

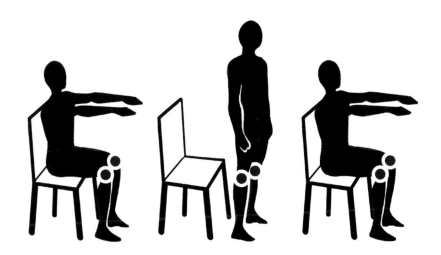

## SIT TO STAND / STAND TO SIT

Sit in a firm, armless chair with your feet flat on the floor and your arms crossed or loose at your sides, whichever feels more balanced. Slowly stand up, using deliberate, controlled movements, until you are standing up  . Hold for a few seconds, and then slowly sit down again. Repeat this exercise . A firm cushion can be placed on the chair if this move is difficult at first. Tip: Check your knees -- when going up or down, they should never move forward beyond your toes. Use your hands to push a little, if this is very difficult.

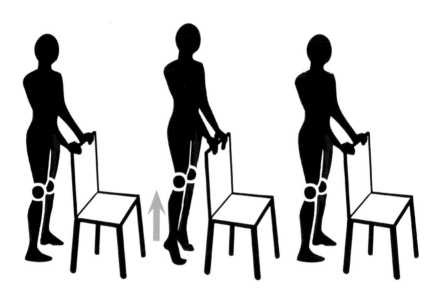

## STANDING HEEL RAISES

This exercise builds calf strength and ankle stability, as well as body coordination and balance. Ankle stability is critical to proper knee alignment.

While standing, raise up on your toes as you lift your heels off the ground.

Lower to the starting position in a slow, controlled manner.

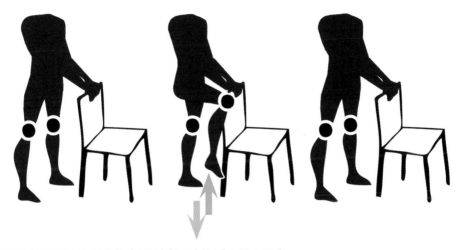

## STANDING MARCHING - SINGLE LEG

While standing old on sturdy chair , draw up one knee toward your chest, your toes pointed up the entire time, set it down on the floor to the original position and then repeat on the other side. Use your arms for support if needed for balance and safety.

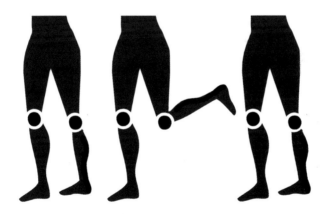

## HAMSTRING CURL

You should feel this exercise at the back of your thigh. Hold on to the back of a chair for balance. Plant your weight onto your supporting leg. Lift the other foot and bring the heel up toward your buttocks. Hold for 3 to 5 seconds. Slowly lower your leg. Repeat and switch sides. Do: Keep your knees close together.

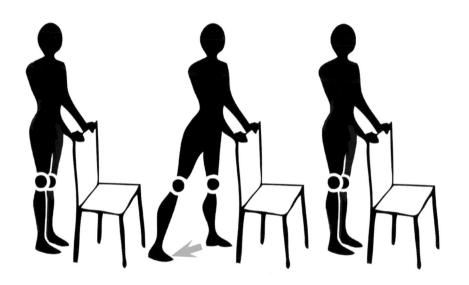

## HIP ABDUCTION - STANDING

While standing, hold on to a sturdy chair, raise your leg out to the side only about 45 degrees. Keep your knee straight and maintain your toes pointed forward the entire time. Slowly take your leg back to the original position then repeat and switch sides.
Use your arms for support if needed for balance and safety.

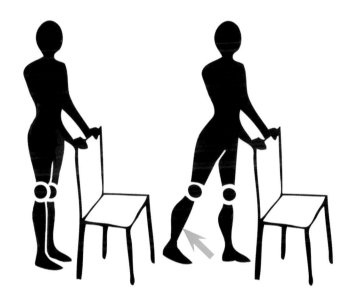

## HIP EXTENSION - STANDING

While standing, hold on to a sturdy chair. Start this exercise by moving one leg back as shown. The movement has to be done slowly and all you need here is about 20 degrees of extension. Maintain your toes pointed forward the entire time. Go back to the original position slowly. Alternate legs and repeat.

Use your arms for support if needed for balance and safety.

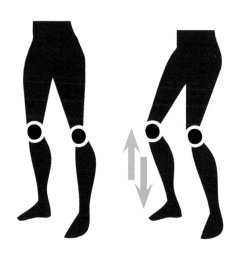

## MINI SQUAT

Start with your feet shoulder-width apart and toes pointed straight ahead. Next, bend your knees to approximately 30 degrees of flexion to perform a mini squat as shown. Then, return to original position.

Knees should bend in line with the 2nd toe and not pass the front of the foot.

Use a chair for support if needed for balance and safety.

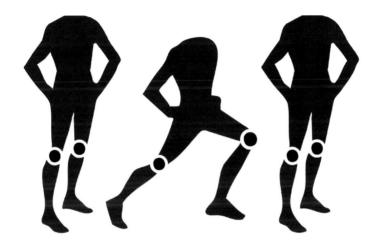

## LUNGE

Start by standing with feet shoulder-width apart. Next, take a step forward and allow your front knee to bend. Your back knee may bend as well. Then, return to original position, or you may walk and take a step forward and repeat with the other leg.

Next we will cover "support"… what you can do to help your knees feel better when they are not functioning properly.

# 8

## SUPPORT

What you will learn in this chapter:

- Most of us will experience knee pain at some point and "Support" is about knowing what to do when this occurs

- Although they aren't cures, topical treatments and support garments can help you feel better and be able to do more, without taking much risk

- One of the most effective topical treatments is menthol

- Menthol comes from the mint and peppermint plants and is one of the most effective "natural" pain relievers

- Although the way menthol works is debated by scientists, it appears to provide pain relief through its cooling effect on nerve endings and interruption of pain signals to the brain

- Compression helps by controlling swelling and giving you a sense of support so that you will continue to use the knee (and knee muscles)

- Compression garments that contain metal or rigid braces are generally not recommended unless you have had a major ligament injury or surgery, because rigid devices take over for the muscles and can lead to muscle weakening

- Over the counter medications can be utilized and can be effective, but can carry significant risks

- When these basic support options are not enough, it is time to consider, prescription medications, injections, and surgical options

If you're experiencing knee pain bad enough that it's interfering with your life, there are some non-invasive "supports" that can give you significant relief.

Although they aren't cures, topical treatments and support garments can help you feel better without taking much risk. As you know, when you feel better you're able to perform more of the activities you love and need to accomplish, plus it will be a whole lot easier to do the physical activity we talked about in Chapter Seven. It keeps you from saying: It hurts - so I'll put this off.

## TOPICAL TREATMENTS

Let's talk first about topical treatments, which are either lotions, creams or gels that are applied on to the skin in the area of concern. Topical treatments have the advantage of being applied right where the pain is and typically have little uptake into the bloodstream. Because of this, there theoretically is less of a chance of undesired side effects or interaction with other medications. Many topicals are available over the counter and there are also some prescription options.

My personal favorite topical preparations contain menthol, in part because I experienced the substantial benefit of a mentholated topical recently when I strained my neck, but also because I have thoroughly investigated topicals (including unscientifically surveying thousands of my patients about their preferences and reviewing available studies). I have concluded that they work. And they work better, with less potential downside than the other types of topicals.

Menthol is one of nature's most soothing and effective chemical compounds. It comes from plants we commonly know as mint and peppermint.

You've probably used a product with menthol at some point in your life, but did you ever stop to think why it feels so good and seems to give such immediate relief?

Although the exact mechanism through which menthol works to relieve pain is not exactly known, menthol is thought to work by promoting temporary numbing around the application site, tricking your brain into perceiving a cooling effect. The cooling sensation relieves the pain you feel by interrupting pain signals that would normally go to the spinal cord and up to the brain.

Menthol also may enhance uptake through the skin of other "anti-inflammatory" ingredients.

Although scientists will continue to study these mechanisms, what you need to know is that:

*"for hundreds of years menthol has been used to relieve pain and suffering throughout the world."*

Many physicial therapists regularly incorporate the use of mentholated products on their patients. Why do they do this?...... because it helps. Interestingly, some people shun topical treatments saying "it only helps a while and then wears off." Is that so bad? If something makes you feel better and is typically very safe, and can be used again and again......how is that a bad thing? Remember, nothing in life is permanent (including life itself) and there are no guarantees with any treatment.

Menthol is typically well tolerated by most adults and is most likely the "safest" over the counter pain reliever sold. However, side effects and allergic reactions are possible with anything. Avoid putting on any mucus membranes (eg. eyes, mouth, nose, genitals) and wash your hands after applying. It should not be applied to irritated skin. Heat lamps, heating pads and bandages should not be utilized at the same time, or there is potential for skin burns. Follow guidance from the label on any product or drug utilized.

## COMPRESSION

Compression is the second part of this dynamic feeling-better duo.

Compression helps by controlling swelling. When you reduce swelling, you reduce pain. Have you ever noticed that many professional athletes – who by definition subject their bodies to excessive amounts of wear and tear – are wearing support devices during their games? Why do you think that is?

Support devices give a *sensation* of support and contribute to general stability without providing rigid support. Because your knee feels supported, you are more likely to use it. Every time you use your knee, your muscles work. And you already know by now how important it is to keep those muscles working.

What I'm not talking about here are support devices like braces that are rigid and contain metal or hinges. Rigid support devices are usually not a good idea unless you've had a major ligament injury or surgery. Why? They "take over" for the muscles and cause them to weaken through lack of use. Employing bracing where it's not necessary is in many cases counterproductive because…

*…Good knee care is all
about strengthening the muscles!*

Compression can be as simple as wrapping an elastic bandage around the knee or wearing a "sleeve." Both are available in drugstores as well as on the internet.

It's important that whatever you choose be comfortable and not bulky or else you won't wear it. And while some people may experience immediate relief, for others it will take time.

When topical treatments and using the support sleeve are still not enough, it may be time to consider over the counter medications.

# OVER THE COUNTER MEDICATIONS

Over-the-counter medications are designed to help further reduce pain or inflammation.

If you're like some of my patients, you might be thinking "A medication is a temporary fix, a patch. Just give me surgery and let's be done with it."

I don't agree with that line of thinking, and here's why (this is my philosophical side, not my doctor side): Life is temporary, and it's about feeling as good as you can with as little risk as possible. Every day is precious. You never know what life holds in store for you, so why not try medication if nothing else has worked. Many times knee pain comes and goes (even though the anatomical problem persists), and if taking some medication for a short time can make that happen, why not?

My conviction is strong that you should resort to surgery only if and when you *really* have to. Not everyone with knee pain or arthritis needs the most invasive treatment. At least not right away. And certainly not until the mind and body have been optimized to have the best possible outcome.

So, what are your non-prescription options? First, always check with your primary care doctor before taking any over-the-counter medication.

*"Just because something is sold over the counter does not mean that it is safe for everyone to take."*

Remember, there is some potential risk with every decision we make. It is amazing how many patients I see that, given their individual situation (eg. medical issues, medications being taken), are regularly using an over the counter medicine that they should not be. They are literally risking their lives every day, and don't even know it. With a little education however, smart decisions can be made. Read the package insert for whatever you choose to take. Discuss with your physician and your pharmacist if there are any interactions with other medications you are taking or issues with health conditions you have. It's also important for your primary doctor to know if you are taking these often so they can monitor you for potential side effects (eg. checking your liver and kidney function with blood tests, monitoring for signs of internal bleeding, etc).

There are two classes of over-the-counter medications typically used to treat knee pain
   1. Acetaminophen
   2. Anti-inflammatories


## ACETAMINOPHEN

Acetaminophen is a non-narcotic pain reliever. The best-known one is Tylenol. It's a fairly safe drug as long as you don't take too much of it (carefully comply with dosage recommendations – more is not better.) In excess it can cause liver damage and even death [24]. It is not appropriate for people with liver disease or people who are heavy users of alcohol. Acetaminophen is also commonly mixed with other medications (eg. cold medicines, allergy medicines, and narcotic pain relievers), so it can be easier than you think to overdose. The FDA has realized this and has decreased the amount allowed in combination pills and manufacturers have changed their labeling to recommend a dose no greater than 3000 mg daily (equal to 6 extra strength 500 mg tablets).

Like most drugs, the data on acetaminophen effectiveness is mixed for treating knee pain and arthritis, but many patients do find it helpful.

## ANTI-INFLAMMATORIES

Anti-inflammatories do what their name implies, they reduce inflammation, but also relieve pain. These are also known as NSAIDs (non-steroidal anti-inflammatory drugs). Popular over-the-counter brands include ibuprofen compounds, such as Motrin and Advil; and naproxen, such as Aleve. Aspirin is also an NSAID.

As we have learned, inflammation is a significant factor in knee pain, so it stands to reason that if you reduce the inflammation, you reduce the pain. The downside of anti-inflammatories is that they have more potential side effects than acetaminophen including stomach upset, ulcers, kidney problems and effects on the heart and blood pressure (cardiovascular system). They also can thin the blood, so patients on blood thinners like warfarin (brand name Coumadin), clopidogrel (brand name Plavix) and many others should not take these. People do bleed and even die from NSAID's every year, so be careful if you choose to use these. Each year approximately 103,000 people are hospitalized and there are 16,500 deaths related to NSAID use [25].

Nevertheless, NSAID's can help many people relieve pain, have less stiffness and better quality of life. So for many people without significant risk factors, they are worth a try.

Now we've looked at all the most basic and safest support options for dealing with knee injury and pain, and reviewed over the counter medications available and their risks. If there are still issues with your knees that are interfering with quality of life and ability to function, turn the page to read about what doctors have to offer.........prescription medications, injections, and surgery.

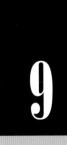

# WHEN IT GETS BAD

What you will learn in this chapter:

- Finding the right doctor requires asking for recommendations from your primary care doctor, nurses, physical therapists, friends and family, and carefully researching the doctor's credentials

- When you seek medical intervention for your pain, the doctor can offer various treatment options depending on your situation. These include medications, injections and surgery

- For your doctor's appointment, you should be prepared to answer questions about your problem and also be ready to ask your doctor questions that will help educate you about your particular situation and suggested treatment options

- You should resort to surgery only when you have exhausted all other possibilities

- Some surgeries are done arthroscopically with small incisions and a camera

- Knee replacement is an open surgery where implants are inserted

- Not all knee replacement surgery is total replacement. Sometimes only part of the knee needs to be replaced

- With complete knee replacement, it can take up to 12 to 18 months for full recovery

- The success of any knee surgery depends on many variables including the surgeon's skill, the type of replacement parts used and individual patient factors

OK. So you've done everything you've read about in this book. You've learned about knees. You're exercising. You've lost weight. You're eating a nutritious diet, and you've given the right supplements plenty of time to work. You're supporting your knee in order to reduce the pain and inflammation and are following the healthiest lifestyle you possibly can.

Despite all this, your knee is still keeping you from doing the things you love to do.

What now?

It's time to make an appointment with an orthopedic surgeon. I assure you not all knee doctors are created equal, so it is worth your time and effort to seek out a knowledgable and experienced surgeon.

The following information can help you find the right doctor:

# CHOOSING A DOCTOR

- Request a recommendation from your primary care physician. He or she knows who the top doctors are in your area. A good question to ask is: "If your (wife/husband) needed knee surgery, to whom would you send them?"

- Ask friends and family members who have had knee problems to recommend someone they like and trust. Was the doctor easy to talk to? Did the doctor's recommendations make sense for their particular situation? Do they have any regrets about going to that doctor?

- One of the best sources of referrals can be nurses who work at the hospital with the surgeons and physical therapists that work with post-operative patients. These practitioners see the results of the different surgeons in a community and are likely to give unbiased recommendations based on what they see.

- Look for a doctor who is board certified by the American Board of Orthopaedic Surgery (ABOS.ORG) and is a Fellow in the American Academy of Orthopaedic Surgeons (AAOS. ORG).  For younger people with "sports" injuries, additional board certification in sports medicine is desirable as well as membership in the American Orthopaedic Society for Sports Medicine (SPORTSMED.ORG).  For people considering knee replacement, look for membership in the American Association of Hip and Knee Surgeons (AAHKS.ORG).  While none of these are guarantees of excellence, physicians with these certifications have had to pass rigorous testing and evaluations to ensure a basic level of competency.

- Find out in advance if your insurance plan is accepted by a physician you are considering seeing. Don't hesitate to use "out of network" benefits if that is what is needed to find the best physician. It is your health and your future, if you have to spend a little extra to see the best, then do it!

- If surgery is recommended, never feel bad about seeking an independent second opinion if desired. Surgery, as we have discussed, presents risks and, in the case of total knee replacement, can involve a lengthy recovery.  Make sure you need it!

I know. You're worried that the doctor will tell you that you need surgery, and you've heard the stories, maybe from a friend, of a knee operation that didn't work out too well. Relax, there are some potentially helpful medical therapies worth trying long before the dreaded "S" word becomes significant.

## BEFORE YOUR APPOINTMENT

You can prepare in advance for getting the most out of the initial doctor's appointment by being prepared to answer the questions below, which your doctor is likely to ask you:

- When did you first notice discomfort in your knee?
- Are you aware of any way you might have injured your knee?
- How frequently do you get symptoms? Only occasionally when you do certain activities or all the time?
- If only during certain activities, which ones?
- On a scale of 1-10 with 10 being the worst, how bad do you consider the pain to be most of the time?
- Are there things you do that definitely make the pain get worse or get better?

- Are you using any over-the-counter or prescription medications for pain or inflammation?
- Do you take any joint support supplements like glucosamine?
- Is the pain interfering with your quality of life?  Your ability to function and do the things you need to do (eg.  work, sleep, be active)?

And since questions go both directions, you might want to consider having a few questions of your own prepared to ask your physician. For example…

- What do you think could be causing my pain?
- How likely is the problem to go away on its own?
- Is there anything I can do to improve the condition and avoid or postpone the need for surgery?
- What can I be doing to improve the overall health of my knees?
- What kind of test(s) are you recommending for me, and why those?
- What will those tests be able, and unable, to tell you about my condition?
- If you are going to prescribe prescription medication, what can I expect it to do? What are its limitations? Must I take it with food? Is it safe to drive or consume alcohol while on this medication? How long will I be on it before I experience results? Will I have to be on it indefinitely?  What are the risks?
- What activities should I avoid?
- What activities should I be doing on a regular basis?
- Can surgery help?  If so, what are the surgical options?

- What is the chance of success with surgery?
- What are the risks of surgery?
- What are reasonable expectations with each treatment option discussed?

When you seek medical intervention for your pain, the doctor can offer various treatment options depending on your situation. These include medications, injections and surgery.

## PRESCRIPTION MEDICATIONS

There are prescription versions of anti-inflammatories (NSAIDS) which your doctor might order that are similar in structure and effectiveness to the over-the-counter versions. These include meloxicam, diclofenac, ibuprofen, naproxen, celecoxib, and many others. You may need to try several different ones to determine which works best for you. These medications can improve the quality of your life and make your knee pain bearable enough that that's all you'll need. All the medications of this type though have the same potential risks and side effects including stomach upset, ulcers, kidney issues, cardiovascular effects and bleeding. Close monitoring by your physician is necessary. These should never be taken in combination with each other or combined with over the counter versions of anti-inflammatories. I see a lot of patients who are on a prescription NSAID, that are also taking an over the counter NSAID, and this can be very dangerous and even life threatening. They also should not be taken with any blood thinners for two serious reasons. First, they also can make the blood thinner, increasing risk of serious bleeding. Second, if an ulcer develops while on a blood thinner, death becomes a very serious possibility.

Recently the Food and Drug Administration approved an anti-depressant, duloxetine (Cymbalta) for the treatment of chronic osteoarthritis pain. This approval recognizes the link between arthritis pain and mental health. The results vary from person to person, and can take weeks to months to start working. Its use should be avoided in people taking other antidepressants, thiroidazine, and people with glaucoma. There are a lot of potential interactions and side effects, so be sure to discuss thoroughly with your doctor if you consider taking this medication.

Patients diagnosed with Rheumatoid and other forms of inflammatory arthritis are best managed by a rheumatologist (a physician that specializes in these kinds of problems). There have been numerous special medicines developed which can help control symptoms for many people. Of course, these also have their risks, but in general the medicines available now have dramatically improved the lives of people suffering with these types of arthritis.

You may wonder why I didn't include narcotic pain medications like codeine, hydrocodone, oxycodone and others in my list. Well, that's because those and the other opiates are the worst and most counterproductive treatments a person can use.

I see them as a slippery slope. First, opiates are highly addictive, and second, your body builds up a tolerance to them. Over time you need more and more. Eventually, they simply don't work. At all.

A patient who's a candidate for surgery and taking opiates for pain presents a significant challenge to the surgeon. Pain that results from surgery that is usually controlled short-term by the kind of pain medications the patient has been taking (or less strong pain killing medications) cannot be controlled because the patient already has built up a tolerance to them. In essence, they've "used up" the best pain-fighting weapons we have during a time when they really weren't needed. I end up sending those patients back to their doctors to wean them off the opiates and reset their pain threshold. This takes time, and only then can we have a successful surgical outcome.

## INJECTIONS

Sometimes injections are indicated. The most prevalent injections fall under two general types, corticosteroids and hyaluronic acid. Both only treat symptoms. Neither produces a cure.

Corticosteroids are the most common. Even though there's limited scientific evidence that they are super effective, many patients and doctors swear by them. I see them as a good way to insert a powerful anti-inflammatory into the area of where the pain is.

That being said, caution is required in their use. In large doses or used too often, corticosteroids can be destructive to cartilage and bone. For diabetics, a cortisone injection can raise the blood sugar levels.

I generally recommend a single shot of cortisone for most knee problems that have not improved with other methods described. I don't have an explanation, but often times despite what is going on inside the knee, the injection just helps the patient feel significantly better. Sometimes this lasts, sometimes not.

Hyaluronic acid is another option but an even more controversial one, because there's recent evidence that it doesn't help as much as had been previously thought (we talked about how hard it is to prove something is effective in Chapter 5). In fact, the American Academy of Orthopedic Surgery recently recommended against its use in knees, concluding that it is not effective, despite some studies that show otherwise. The shots are expensive, must be given multiple times and may or may not be covered by insurance.

These injections are sometimes known as "gel shots" or "rooster shots." They're called "gel shots" because it's believed the compound may beef up the thick synovial fluid of the knee that gets thinner as people age. They're nicknamed "rooster shots" because some are made from processed chicken or rooster combs.

I have seen these shots help many people including family members. I continue to use them when appropriate because it is a "natural" substance, rarely has adverse effects and, I believe, helps about 2 out of 3 people who get it. Now it is not a cure and does not regrow cartilage, but it is still an option to try prior to considering surgery for many patients.

Two of the newest therapies are yet even more controversial and are not commonly used because they are considered experimental (and not covered by insurance). Platelet rich plasma (PRP), which uses the patient's own blood, and stem cells fall under the category of "regenerative medicine."

I'm mentioning them here because they've been in the media a lot lately. Only time will tell if they become safe and effective treatments for knee problems. I just don't think there is enough safety data or reports of effectiveness to recommend considering these at this time.

**And finally, it's time to address the possibility of surgery.**

When you make a decision about anything in life – even getting in your car and driving to the grocery store - you must keep in mind that risk is involved. Everything you do is a calculated risk, most times with overwhelming odds in your favor. However, things can and do go wrong. Just as car accidents sometimes happen, surgeries occasionally don't turn out the way they were intended. We quoted a statistic earlier in the book that around 1 in 5  patients receiving a total knee replacement were disappointed by the results. Even though my surgical patients have a higher satisfaction rate than that with the use of new techniques and technologies, it's not something I take lightly when deciding on the best course of action. Nor should you.

It's important to weigh the potential benefits against the risk, which is what I do every single day in my practice. The patient's age, physical condition, lifestyle and goals are all factors that make every case different. Let's say I have two patients with a torn ACL ligament. One is 20 and very athletic and the other is 50 and works in an office. I'm more likely to recommend consideration of surgery on the younger one because the younger one most likely has a healthy knee, will be higher demand on the knee, and needs the surgery to protect the knee and make it last as long as possible. The 50 year old, by contrast, most likely already has degeneration of the knee and repairing the issue with the ligament is not going to stop that.  The risk of the surgery in the 50 year old's case is not worth the small, if any, potential benefit.

Like me, other orthopedic surgeons will also have finely-honed practices for deciding the appropriate course of action. Once you've chosen a surgeon, I suggest you let him or her proceed the way they deem best, and trust their judgment. If you don't trust their judgment, find a surgeon whose judgment you do trust.

That being said, it certainly doesn't hurt to be a bit more educated about knee surgeries. In general, we will discuss the common operations performed (there are lots of operations performed on the knee but a complete discussion is beyond the scope of this book). The goal here is not to tell you everything you need to know about the surgeries (there are plenty of books and websites about that which you should also investigate), the goal is to give you some of the information you need when considering surgery to make an educated decision. It is, after all, your body and your life.

*"Fortunately, the overwhelming majority of patients who undergo knee surgery will have a good or great outcome."*

Nevertheless, just like driving your car (in the US alone tens of thousands die each year in motor vehicle accidents), surgery involves risk. The serious risks and complications from surgery (eg. infection, loss of limb, heart attack, stroke, pulmonary embolism and death) are not common statistically, unless they happen to you. With that said, if you have done everything possible to avoid surgery and you are not better, than doing nothing also has risk. Chronic knee pain can cause depression, inactivity and weight gain. All of these can also be devastating for your general health and well being. So don't be so scared of surgery that you don't get it if you need it. Everyone will have their own set point of when they decide. If you have put into place the lifestyle changes discussed in this book, you have already decreased your chances of complications and improved your chances of a good outcome with surgery.

# ARTHROSCOPIC SURGERY

Arthroscopic surgery of the knee is a minimally invasive way of addressing problems within the joint including meniscal tears, loose pieces of cartilage or bone, and ligament ruptures. It involves making a few stab wounds around the knee and inserting a camera and some instruments to do the work that needs to be done while the surgeon watches on a TV as he works. In an otherwise healthy knee (typically someone less than 40 years old), it can be an excellent way to treat a ligament injury or isolated meniscal tear. However, more than half of the approximately 1 million arthroscopic surgeries performed annually are in knees with meniscal tears and degenerative joint disease. Most recent studies reveal that with a meniscal tear in the presence of degeneration of the joint (osteoarthritis), physical therapy and non-operative management can be just as effective as intervention with arthroscopic surgery. About eighty percent of people with osteoarthritis of the knee will have a diagnosable meniscal tear if an MRI is done, and many of these people have no symptoms and do not need treatment.

In my office, there is hardly a week that goes by that I don't see several people requesting second opinions that had an arthroscopic knee surgery in the past few months or years and are wondering why they are not better. My surgeon told me he "cleaned out the arthritis." I explain to them that arthritis is something that is missing (cartilage, that spongy substance we learned about in chapter 1) and that no surgeon can clean out something that is already missing. The surgeon can sometimes smooth out the rough edges of cartilage or torn meniscus which may improve the mechanical symptoms (locking and catching with pain that occurs with movement). So how do I know if arthroscopic surgery is indicated or can help? On the next page are some general guidelines as a good starting point to discuss with your surgeon.

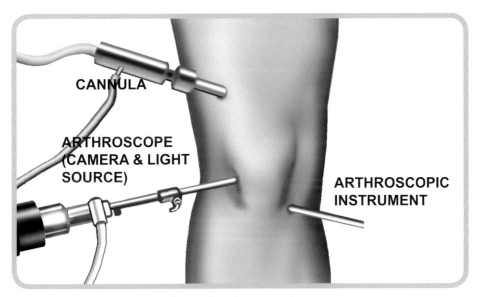

Illustration of arthroscopic surgery

- If the knee is arthritic and pain is the main issue, avoid arthroscopic surgery. Utilize the lifestyle approach described in this book and the other non-operative means mentioned. If not successful, consider partial or total knee replacement surgery.

- If there is a meniscal tear, the knee is arthritic and pain is the main issue, try and avoid arthroscopic surgery. Utilize the lifestyle approach described in this book and the other non-operative means mentioned. If not successful, consider partial or total knee replacement surgery.

- If there is a meniscal tear and the main symptoms are mechanical (eg. locking, catching, buckling) in association with pain, and the knee has minimal to no arthritis, then arthroscopic surgery should be considered.

- If there is a meniscal tear with just pain and no mechanical symptoms in an otherwise healthy joint, consider a trial of non-operative treatment. Remember, the surgery does not fix the meniscus (except rarely in some children and young athletes). The meniscus is just trimmed away. If surgery is not performed and the pain subsides, you can just live with the tear and may very well forget you ever had it.

- If the Anterior Cruciate Ligament (ACL) and/or other important ligaments are ruptured and you are young (less than forty), and the knee is healthy, it may be beneficial to reconstruct the ligament so surgery should be considered.

- Once you are over 40 with an ACL tear and/or other ruptured ligaments and the knee is otherwise healthy, the decision to reconstruct becomes less clear, particularly for someone who is not an athlete. The risks and benefits should be considered, as it might make more sense to take other measures designed to create stability and rehabilitate the muscle around the knee. Once the knee is arthritic, the ACL tear is no longer relevant and the lifestyle approach should be tried. Knee replacement procedures should be considered if needed.

There are other arthroscopic and non-arthoscopic surgeries that attempt to preserve the knee, like cartilage repair and osteotomies (cutting the bones and realigning), that may be worth considering in individual cases. At some point in the future we may be able to regrow cartilage more effectively and restore the surface of the joint. But at this time, for the bulk of people with degenerative knees, there are only two reasonable surgical options.......Partial Knee Replacement (PKR) and Total Knee Replacement (TKR).

## KNEE REPLACEMENT

A knee replacement is actually not a great name. It implies that the entire knee is removed and replaced with a large mechanical device. More accurately, what is done, is just the surfaces of the joint (either part or all of it) and a few millimeters of bone are replaced with metal and plastic implants. Most of the surrounding structures (the muscle, ligaments, tendons, bones, etc.) remain intact.

You may remember that the knee has three parts: the medial (inside), lateral (outside), and patellofemoral (behind the kneecap). One, two, or all three parts of the knee can degenerate. If only one or two parts of the knee are affected, it is possible to replace only those parts.

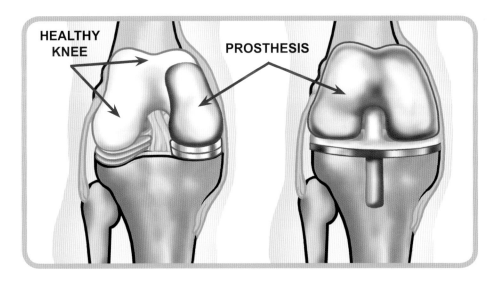

PARTIAL KNEE REPLACEMENT VS. TOTAL KNEE REPLACEMENT

It is worth it to consider this option if that is the case. Many times patients just say "if it is broke, just replace the whole thing." But if one tire on your car is worn out from being out of alignment and the other three have a little wear but plenty of tread left, the same person wouldn't usually say "just replace all four." It goes back to one of the fundamental concepts in this book......do not do more than you need to do.

## There are several potential advantages
## to a partial replacement.

- A partial replacement fixes the part that is bad and leaves behind the others that are ok.

- It is a smaller surgery than a complete replacement, so possibly has less risk.

- It is less invasive and usually recovery is quicker.

- It leaves your knee feeling more like your natural knee with better range of motion.

- It is conservative and doesn't burn bridges for the future. If it doesn't work, you can always do a TKR. If you go right to TKR and it doesn't work or you are not happy with it, there is no going back to a PKR.

## There are some potential disadvantages
## to a partial replacement:

Parts of the knee are left behind that could become arthritic and ultimately cause pain (this is why patient selection and the experience of your surgeon are critical).

Early results may indicate a slightly higher failure rate than with full replacement (but more recent studies indicate excellent long term outcomes at 10 to 15 years, nearly comparable to TKR).

The procedure is not helpful in cases of rheumatoid and other forms of inflammatory arthritis.

Total knee replacement is one of the most time tested surgical procedures having been performed for more than 40 years. While it is a major surgical procedure, it improves the lives of hundreds of thousands of people annually with over 90 percent experiencing a dramatic reduction in pain. The number of people undergoing TKR is a testament to its success. Currently over 600,000 TKR's are performed in the US annually and that number is projected to exceed 3 million by the year 2030.

So if TKR is so great, then why not just get it? Why waste time with all these lifestyle changes and medications?

Surgery involves risk (and in rare cases these can be very serious), but the biggest risk (looking at percentages) appears to be the risk of not being satisfied with the outcome.

Although most people will admit the surgery helped with pain, many (15 to 39 percent in published studies) are NOT satisfied with the outcome of the surgery. Some people still have pain after surgery.

The point of this discussion is not to scare people out of surgery if they need it. I am, after all, a knee replacement surgeon and TKR is the most common operation I perform. The surgery has helped millions of people resume active, pain free lifestyles. The goal here is to make sure you need it and, if you do need it, to minimize risk and improve outcomes.

The success of any knee replacement surgery, including yours, will depend on several variables: the surgeon's technique, the implant used (some fit certain people better than others) and patient factors.

The surgeon's technique is an important factor. This includes the way the surgery is performed, as well as how you are managed before and after the surgery. A doctor can be an excellent surgeon and install the device correctly, but if your pain is not managed properly and you are not given the physical and psychological support you need, it may negatively effect your outcome. The instrumentation surgeons use to implant knee replacements continues to improve with technology, as well as our techniques for managing pain. The research you do in selecting the "right" surgeon using the tips above will go a long way to ensuring you select an excellent surgeon that utilizes all the latest advancements. It is important to find a surgeon that regularly performs TKR. Studies show that a surgeon's outcomes improve when they perform greater than 50 TKR's per year.

The implant chosen can also have a role in the success of the surgery. The goal of the implant is to create a knee that feels natural and as close to your knee as possible. As patients' expectations have risen, the companies that manufacture TKR's have responded with improved design of implants. In the early stages of TKR, companies offered devices in very limited sizes. With the recognition that people come in different shapes and sizes, implant companies have increased their offerings making right and left implants, gender specific implants, and increasing the numbers of sizes available. It is now even possible to create patient specific knees, a device made for each patient that is sized and shaped exactly like the patient's own knee (disclosure.....I have helped design and consult for the company that manufactures these). The potential reward of new technology is that it may make the surgery easier to go through, improve patient satisfaction with the procedure and possibly increase longevity of the device. The potential risk is that the devices are not as time tested as established devices. It is important to realize that no implant (or person) lasts forever. When we look at large numbers of TKRs done worldwide, they tend to fail at a rate of 1% per year. So 90% will last 10 years and 80% will last 20 years. Fortunately, they can usually be redone if they fail.

Patient factors, in my opinion, have the largest impact on the success of TKR. If the success of the surgery depends on minimizing risk and complications, and the patient is the one that judges the satisfaction, then there is a lot the patient can do to influence these variables.

Things YOU can do to ensure the best possible result after TKR:

Educate yourself. Learn as much as you can about knee replacement so you can take the anxiety out of the procedure and know what to expect. Have reasonable expectations. Knee replacement, despite recent techniques and "less invasive" approaches, is still a big surgery. Most people are functioning and back to a normal life within a few weeks, but it can take 1 to 2 years to achieve the final outcome. Don't be disappointed if you don't feel amazing 6 weeks or even 3 months post-operatively.

Do not go into surgery obese. Obesity increases your chance of developing an infection and other serious complications. The odds of mechanical failures also increase due to the additional stress placed on your bone and the implant.

Eat right and don't smoke. Proper nutrition plays an important role in creating healthy bones, muscles, tendons, nerves, blood vessels and skin. Smoking seriously deteriorates all these structures. If you smoke, DO NOT consider knee replacement until you quit.

Exercise. Do this before and after, with or without the help of a physical therapist. The better shape you are in going into surgery, the easier time you will have after. The more flexible your joints are before also has a great impact on how the TKRs bend and function after. Don't stop exercising. Just because you "recover" doesn't mean you shouldn't continue to keep your muscles strong. The muscles need to support your knee implant just as they supported your own knee.

Learn support techniques. It is important to learn how to manage and deal with pain. Many people still have some pain after surgery. Putting in place some simple and effective techniques to manage this can go a long way to ensuring a good outcome.

If these things sound familiar to you after reading this book, it is because they are. They are the same foundation proposed in chapters 4 through 8 for creating a healthy and happy knee. Knee surgeries fix mechanical problems, but do not create knee health. That can only be accomplished by incorporating the principles of education, nutrition, fitness, and support into a lifestyle.

# 10

## CONCLUSION

After reading through this book you should be very well prepared to take care of your knees before any problems become serious, to do everything you can on your own to get your knees as healthy as possible if they're not at their best, and to be an informed patient capable of forging a powerful, therapeutic relationship with your doctor.

You know about knee anatomy, what can cause knee problems and the limitations of modern medicine.

You know about the concepts of risk, how to determine if a treatment is effective, and what to expect with each stage of life.

And most important, you know about the need for lifestyle change and the four very powerful ways you can take charge of your knee health.

Let's just do a quick recap of those ways:

- Educating yourself about the knees
- Managing your weight, eating right and utilizing supplements known to promote knee health
- Doing regular, sensible exercise
- Accessing support options including topicals and compression garments to give you relief and knowing when to seek further treatments

You also know that while surgery may ultimately be the "answer," there are many conservative, traditional and non-traditional therapies you can - and should - try first. Surgery, as I have said, is not for everyone and is never without risk. However, surgery can and does help most people when it gets bad, as long as the appropriate foundation for a good outcome (see above) is in place.

Getting and keeping your knees healthy can go a long way toward providing you with a rich life made possible by being able to do the things you love, well into your later years.

That being said, I challenge you to take charge of your knees now that you are empowered with ways to do just that.

Are you ready? Get started today. You have nothing to lose (except maybe some weight) and everything to gain.

# References

1 *N Engl J Med* 2008; 359:1097-1107

2 *N Engl J Med*. 2002 Jul 11;347(2):81-8

3 *Clin Orthop Relat Res*. 2010 Jan;468(1):57-63

4 *Clin Orthop Relat Res*. 2006 Nov;452:35-43

5 *Orthopedics*. 2010 Feb;33(2):76-80

6 *Mayo Clin Proc*. 2013;88(8):790–798

7 *Arthritis*. 2012;2012:504189

8 *Arthritis Rheum* 2008;59(9):1207–1213

9 *Trends Endocrinol Metab*. 2013 Sep;24(9):431-41

10 *Ann Rheum Dis*. 2007 Jan;66(1):18-22

11 *J Arthroplasty*. 2012 Oct;27(9):1690-1695

12 *Am J Sports Med*. 2012 Dec;40(12):2872-8

13 http://www.mayoclinic.com/health/glucosamine/NS_patient-glucosamine/DSECTION=evidence

14 http://www.nlm.nih.gov/medlineplus/druginfo/natural/807.html

15 http://www.nlm.nih.gov/medlineplus/druginfo/natural/662.html

16 *J Altern Complement Med*. 2009 Aug;15(8):891-7

17 *Phytother Res*. 2012 Nov;26(11):1719-25

18 *N Engl J Med* 2013; 368:1675-1684

19 *Osteoarthritis Cartilage*. 2011;19(S1):S145-S146

20 *Adv Exp Med Biol*. 2007;595:105-25

21 *Phytother Res*. 2013 Jul 6. doi: 10.1002/ptr.5025. [Epub ahead of print]

22 *Annals of Internal Medicine* 2012; 157(9): 632-644

23 *Arch Intern Med*. 1999;159(19):2349-2356

24 http://www.fda.gov/drugs/drugsafety/ucm239821.htm

25 *N Engl J Med* 1999;340:1888-1899

For further information on the research supporting
EDUCATION4KNEES visit:
www.EDUCATION4KNEES.com/science